The Positive Psychology
of Personal Transformation

James Garbarino

The Positive Psychology of Personal Transformation

Leveraging Resilience for Life Change

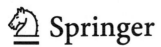 Springer

James Garbarino
Department of Psychology
Center for the Human Rights of Children
Loyola University Chicago
1032 N. Sheridan Rd.
Chicago, IL 60660
USA
jgarbar@luc.edu

ISBN 978-1-4419-7743-4   e-ISBN 978-1-4419-7744-1
DOI 10.1007/978-1-4419-7744-1
Springer New York Dordrecht Heidelberg London

Printed on acid-free paper

Springer is part of Springer Science+Business Media (www.springer.com)

Preface

The miracle is not to walk on water. The miracle is to walk on the green earth, dwelling deeply in the present moment and feeling truly alive.

Thich Nhat Hanh [1]

December 2008, found me facing the discovery that my heart was beating at 125 beats per minute all the time, rather than its normal rate of 70 per minute, and doing so erratically; I was suffering from atrial fibrillation. This explained the exhaustion I had been experiencing for several months. Many tests and medications later, on March 2, 2009, I found myself in the hospital, less than 24 hours away from open heart surgery. Tests conducted by my cardiologist indicated that the heart rate problem was related to the fact that a valve in my heart was leaking seriously (about a 3.5 on a four point scale of severity).

This made it three congenital heart defects that I carried around. Fourteen years earlier I has discovered that one of the two bundles of nerves that led to my heart was not functioning – and presumably never had. This meant that instead of each ventricle of my heart having its own bundle of nerves to control the firing of its muscles, both had to rely on the one functioning bundle (which meant impulses traveled down in to the left ventricle and then jumped over to the right). But further testing showed my heart seemed to have adjusted without detectable damage. The doctor said I might one day need a pacemaker to help compensate for the bundle blockage.

Then 6 years ago I was having chest pains and it turned out I had a blocked artery coming from and servicing my heart. This too appeared to be a congenital defect – the artery came out of the wrong place, connected to the wrong side of my heart, and had "kinked" like a hose, causing the blockage. A procedure to open the blocked artery and keep it open by implanting a wire mesh "stent" seemed to take care of that. But it did increase the risk of having a stroke.

Now here I was spending that first Monday night in March in the hospital in advance of surgery Tuesday morning to repair my leaking valve, wondering if this third congenital "strike" would put me out, and knowing that even if successful, the surgery would mean 8–10 weeks of painful recuperation. To his credit, the heart surgeon on the case repeated some of the tests before opening me up. The results indicated that my valve, though still leaking, was no longer as bad as it had been only weeks earlier when the previous round of tests was completed, perhaps because the medications I was taking had slowed my heart down to a normal level and this permitted the valve to move from a 3.5 to a 1.5 on the leak scale. So I left the hospital the next morning without facing the small chance of dying in the surgery, without a massive scar on my chest, and without having to face at least 8 weeks of painful recuperation and the risk of various complications.

The same year that I did not have the surgery, about 650,000 others did. About 650 died, and nearly 40,000 had serious complications, including strokes [2]. My roommate that Monday night in the hospital had had the surgery two months earlier and was back for his third hospitalization because of complications. He was gracious enough to share my good feeling about being spared, but it was clear that what he had gone through had destabilized him psychologically. We talked about how the surgery had changed his life in ways he never anticipated – most of the worse, but some for the better.

I left the hospital the next day thinking about Thich Nhat Hanh's words about the miracle of walking the green Earth and what my hospital roommate had said about the "for the better." It was easy for me to be happy about my fate that day, of course. I was permitted to continue walking freely on the Earth. But I left reflecting on how it was that my roommate could find anything positive in *his* situation. For days after my release I thought about what it took to find the positive in human suffering as Buddhists and Christians alike are taught. I thought long and hard about what role being positive played in my own life – before, during, and now after my brush with open heart surgery. And, as I went about my business – being with my family, reflecting on my experience, and working at my job as a college professor – I realized I was ready to write this book, a book about what I have learned about the meaning of "being positive" in the face of the human reality of suffering and eventual and inevitable death.

I discerned that in six decades of living I had come to see in myself and in the world around me the quest for a spiritual appreciation of the great opportunity that being alive offers, absolutely and without expectations of comfort, pleasure, and worldly success. I experienced a renewed sense of the gift I have been given by my encounters with Buddhism and my core Christian identity. And I was ready to bring to bear my professional experiences as a psychologist in service of this quest.

While "pop psychology" has long focused upon positive themes of self-understanding, human potential, empowerment, and assertiveness, most scientific psychology in America has long and mostly focused upon either the neutral processes of mental functioning (such as memory, cognition) or the negative developments that plague human lives: studying them, preventing them, treating them. In recent years, however, scientific psychology has developed a new focus on the positive, with an emphasis on thriving, happiness, and fulfillment.

In this sense, it is rejoining the "humanistic" psychology that emerged in the 1950s and 1960s but was soon marginalized or abandoned by mainstream scientific psychology. This was in part for its methodological shortcomings, and in part for its attention to topics then thought to be inherently "unscientific" such as spirituality, meaning, and higher purpose. This trend continued until humanistic psychology was "rescued" by psychologist–researchers Martin Seligman, Mihaly Csikszentmihalyi, and their colleagues and followers.

The development of positive psychology in the scientific mainstream in some ways parallels the history of psychoanalysis in the sense that some of its concepts (e.g., "Freudian Slips" and "the unconscious"), which were dismissed as "unscientific" by behaviorist psychologists in the 1950s and 1960s, have been rehabilitated in more recent neuropsychological research that finds a biological basis for these concepts in modern brain research.

Students of positive psychology have taken many of the ideas in humanistic psychology and given them scientific credibility as a movement that is most closely associated with the work of Martin Seligman, who made it the theme of his presidency of the American Psychological Association in 1998. His book *Authentic Happiness: Using the New Positive Psychology to Realize Your Potential for Lasting Fulfillment* was a notable milestone, a lovely blend of scientific research, practical suggestions, and highly effective anecdotes [3]. Others have followed suit – e.g., Daniel Gilbert's 2007 book *Stumbling on Happiness*, Ben Shahar's 2007 book *Happier: Learn the Secrets to Daily Joy and Lasting Fulfillment*, and Fred Bryant and Joseph Veroff's book on *Savoring: A New Model of Positive Experience* [4–6].

Seligman offered three "pillars" of positive psychology: the study of positive emotion, the study of positive traits (strengths, virtues, and abilities such as intelligence and athleticism), and the study of positive institutions that support the virtues, and thus the positive emotions. From these comes a focus on three themes. The first is the "life of enjoyment." By this he refers to efforts to understand how and why people enjoy what in an earlier era would have been called "the simple pleasures of life" – their social relationships, hobbies, and other activities that entertain them, the satisfaction of ordinary living. The second theme concerns the "life of engagement." The focus here is on investigating the beneficial results that come from giving oneself over to some pursuit. The sense of confidence, competence, achievement, and timelessness that comes from giving your all to some activity has long been recognized as important for a sense of well being, but it has become the topic of formal study most notably in the work of Mihaly Csikszentmihalyi and his concept of "flow" [7].

The third focal point identified by Seligman is the "life of affiliation." Here the focus is on how being part of a bigger picture generates happiness through meaningfulness, the sense of being worthwhile that comes from contributing to things beyond one's narrow slice of the larger picture in human existence, the things that endure beyond the momentary ups and downs of an individual human life. These include building institutions, preserving natural resources, helping improve the human condition, and creating culture [8].

While this movement to positive psychology is "news" for mainstream scientific psychology, it is not without its historical origins. If one wishes to name those responsible for focusing on and conceptualizing positive themes in psychological development, perhaps the best classic voices are the humanistic psychologists of the 1950s and 1960s – most notably Abe Maslow, Carl Rogers, and Erich Fromm [9–11].

Joining them have been the many students of spirituality that I have encountered (many of them Buddhists) who have offered up their voices – e.g., French-born Tibetan Buddhist monk Matthieu Ricard, who, in collaboration with American psychologist Daniel Goleman, wrote *Happiness: A Guide to Developing Life's Most Important Skill* in 2007, the Dalai Lama's 1998 *The Art of Happiness: A Handbook for Living*, and the prolific Vietnamese Buddhist monk Thich Nhat Hanh, who in 2007 offered *Two Treasures: Buddhist Teachings on Awakening and True Happiness* (among so many others) [12–14].

The resurgence of positivity in mainstream psychology even owes a debt of intellectual gratitude to some psychologists whose origins lie in a psychoanalytic perspective, such as Erik Erikson and Robert White, whose concepts of mastery and challenge tap positive veins in the human psyche rather than just focusing on the classical Freudian effort to deal with negative drives. Indeed, we can trace the very concept of positive psychology to Maslow's 1954 book *Motivation and Personality* [9].

As a group, these psychologists focused on positive themes such as Maslow's "actualization," Rogers' "unconditional personal regard," Fromm's "biophilia" (love for humanity and nature), Erikson's "generativity" (building something positive in life beyond oneself), and White's "effectance motivation" (which posited a source of energy for ego that was independent of classical Freudian "negative" drive reduction) [9, 15–17]. This affirmation of the human potential for all that is good and beautiful and meaningful and spiritually uplifting has provided the core of humanistic psychology for more than half a century, even though it rested upon and generated little good science. And its adherents have labored on in workshops, books, conferences, and journals mostly treated as an eccentricity by mainstream psychology. At best it has been given lip service in reviews of "the history of psychology" that are offered to students in much the same way that pre-Einstein physics is taught to undergraduate students.

When I was in graduate school at Cornell University in the early 1970s humanistic psychology was very much on the periphery, at best considered a "Third Force" (with behaviorist and psychoanalytic concepts being considered the first two, and this latter approach itself largely discredited and marginalized in mainstream psychology). Indeed, with the rise to preeminence of "behaviorist" psychology in the 1950s and 1960s, "cognitive" psychology in the 1970s and "neuropsychology" in the 1980s, humanistic psychology seemed ever more marginalized, confined to the "softer" domains of "self-improvement" books and workshops that were often derided as "touchy feel" by those who considered themselves practitioners of "psychological science." But with the leadership offered by Martin Seligman's advocacy for positive psychology, the themes addressed by the classic Humanistic Psychologists have found new life as credible topics for serious study and as a source of important explanatory concepts.

This book follows in this revived tradition but with an appreciation for the ultimate value of spiritual exploration in understanding the fundamental human issues addressed by positive psychology. I use my own life experiences as a context for demonstrating the power of positive and humanistic psychology to join with spiritual exploration and practices to help make sense of the human condition. These experiences include my professional activities understanding risk and resilience in war zones, on death row, in child abuse cases, in refugee camps, and as a consultant to a wide range of human service, child welfare, and educational institutions. And, they draw upon my personal experiences as a spouse, as a father, as a citizen, as a companion for dogs, as a world traveler, and perhaps most importantly, as a spiritual seeker. Each explores issues of meaningfulness through reflection on how my own life experiences have highlighted issues dealt with by positive psychology:

- How human relationships with dogs shed light on the core issues of human potential.
- How the costs and benefits of obliviousness are evident in my experience of growing up in the 1950s, and how this sheds light on the need for self-awareness in children and adults.
- How meeting the challenge of trauma reveals some of the most important issues in discovering the origins of "meaningfulness" in human experience.
- How the opposite of trauma is to be found in the positive experience of "transformational grace."
- How narcissism as a cultural and psychological phenomenon in modern life calls for an approach that might be called the "positive death of the self" in favor of the development of the soul.
- How an exploration of the meaning of "living an 'extraordinary' life" brings together the core insights of positive psychology and spiritual development.

This book then is a journey within a journey, and as the classic Chinese proverb tells us, the only way to being such a long journey is with the first step.

Chicago, IL   James Garbarino

References

1. Hanh, T.H. (1990) Peace is every step. New York, NY. Bantam.
2. http://www.nlm.nih.gov/medlineplus.
3. Seligman, M. (2004) Authentic happiness: Using the new positive psychology to realize your potential for lasting fulfillment. New York, NY: Free Press.
4. Gilbert, D. (2007) Stumbling on happiness. New York, NY: Vintage.
5. Ben-Shahar, T. (2007) Happier: Learn the secrets to daily joy and lasting fulfillment. New York, NY: McGraw-Hill
6. Bryant, F. and Veroff, J. Savoring: A new model of positive experience. New Jersey, NJ: Erlbaum.
7. Csikszentmihalyi, M. (2008) Flow: The psychology of optimal experience. New York, NY: Harper Perennial Classics.
8. Seligman, M. (2004) Authentic happiness: Using the new positive psychology to realize your potential for lasting fulfillment. New York, NY: Free Press.
9. Maslow, A. (1954) Motivation and personality. New York, NY: HarperCollins.
10. Rogers, C. (1980) A way of being. New York, NY: Mariner Books.
11. Fromm, E. (1963) The art of loving. New York, NY: Bantam.

12. Ricard, M. and Goleman, D. (2007) Happiness: A guide to developing life's most important skill. Boston: Little, Brown and Company.
13. Lama, D. (2009) The art of happiness: A handbook for living. New York, NY: Penguin.
14. Hanh, T.N. (2007) Two treasures: Buddhist teachings on awakening. True happiness. Berkely, CA: Parallex Press.
15. Fromm, E. (1963) The art of loving. New York, NY; Bantam.
16. Erikson, E. (1995) Childhood and society. New York, NY: Vintage.
17. White, R. (1959) Motivation reconsidered: The concept of competence. Psychological Review. 66, 297–333.

Acknowledgments

I want to thank particularly the group of friendly colleagues who read the first version of this book and encouraged me to finish it: Charles Swadley, Fred Bryant, Donald Gault, and David Crenshaw. And I wish to thank my brother John and Wendy Behary, who helped me through my own process of personal transformation. And finally, I wish to thank Claire Bedard, who has taught me more about love and generosity than anyone else in my life.

About the Author

James Garbarino was the founding Director of the Center for the Human Rights of Children at Loyola University Chicago and is the current Maude C. Clarke Chair in Humanistic Psychology. Before arriving at Loyola, he was Cornell University's Elizabeth Lee Vincent Professor of Human Development and co-director of the Family Life Development Center. He received his bachelor's degree from St. Lawrence University and a doctorate in human development and family studies from Cornell University. From 1985–1994 he was President of the Erikson Institute for Advanced Study in Child Development. Dr. Garbarino has served as a consultant to a wide range of organizations, including the National Committee to Prevent Child Abuse, the National Institute for Mental Health, the American Medical Association, the U.S. Advisory Board on Child Abuse and Neglect, and the Federal Bureau of Investigation. He also serves as an expert witness in criminal and civil cases involving issues of violence and children. Books he has authored or edited include: *Children and the Dark Side of Human Experience, Lost Boys, See Jane Hit: Why Girls Are Growing More Violent and What We Can Do About It*, and *Words Can Hurt Forever: How to Protect Adolescents from Bullying, Harassment, and Emotional Violence*. His work has also been featured in television, magazines, and newspapers, including appearances on "The Today Show," "Dateline," and "Larry King Live." Dr. Garbarino has received numerous awards, including the first C. Henry Kempe Award from the National Conference on Child Abuse and Neglect, Fellow of the American Psychological Association, Spencer Fellow by the National Academy of Education, National Fellow by the Kellogg Foundation, and the President's Celebrating Success Award from the National Association of School Psychologists. He is a former president of the American Psychological Association's Division on Child, Youth and Family Services.

Contents

1   **Walking with Hope and Dharma: Are Dogs Enlightened? Are Humans?** 1

2   **The Costs and Benefits of Obliviousness: Growing Up in the 1950s** 23

3   **Nine Bad Things That Almost Happened, and Many More That Did: Getting to the Other Side of Trauma** 43

4   **What Is the Opposite of Trauma? The Positive Power of Transformational Grace** 65

5   **Can There Ever Be Enough Me? Narcissism and the Positive Death of Self** 81

6   **What Does It Mean to Live an "Extraordinary Life?"** 103

Index 119

Chapter 1
Walking with Hope and Dharma:
Are Dogs Enlightened? Are Humans?

Walking with Hope and Dharma. "Walking" conveys the sense that life is a journey. "Hope" is at the core of Christianity and positive psychology, and in everyday language is the foundation for living amidst the disappointments of life, what Barack Obama has called the "audacity" to believe in a positive path despite the realities that discourage us. In Buddhism, "Dharma" is the teaching that defines, illuminates, and guides us along the path to Enlightenment. These teachings about the nature of self complement my spiritual life as a Christian.

However, in my life, *Walking with Hope and Dharma* is more than this. It is *literally* walking with Hope and Dharma, for Hope and Dharma are the names of my canine companions – 50 pound Black Lab mixes. Most days when I am home, the dogs and I walk three miles at our local state park, along a path and around a small lake. These walks are an important anchor in my life, a time and a place to reflect on life and living. And these walks gave rise to this book, as I reflected on how the concepts of the emerging field of "positive psychology" resonated with my emerging understanding of my spiritual life as a Christian informed by Buddhism.

It's not just the walking, of course. And it's not just about the dogs, either. My relationship with these two dogs is opening my eyes and heart to a better understanding of all the relationships in my life – past and present, canine and human. *Walking With Hope and Dharma* is a reflection on the ups and downs of growing up and aging, the highs and lows of parenthood and marriage, the insights and blockages of self-awareness and insight, and the residue of many extraordinary experiences – in war zones, refugee camps, prisons, schools, and communities around the world – over the six decades of my life. Through all of this dogs have been a constant feature. Dharma and Hope are not the first dogs in my life, but it is possible that they may be the last: I am old enough and they are young enough for me to make this a real possibility.

My baby photo album features my English grandparents' "Kelpie," and the dog my parents had when I was born, "Boots." The photo albums of childhood contain the multiple mutts who came in and out of my life as my parents took dogs in and sent them off for reasons that to this day I sometimes can't fathom. The one dog who came and stayed in my parents' life was Coco – a brown and white mixed breed who loved chocolate (which is now known to be toxic to dogs, but back then people didn't seem to know about such things). She was the emotional mainstay of my family through the 1960s until well after I went off to college and moved out on my own. Home for the summer after my first year in college, I impulsively bought a yellow Lab-mix puppy who at first went by the name "Lady Bird" (then the First Lady to Lyndon Johnson's President), but who soon was renamed "Sam." When I couldn't take the young dog back to college with me my parents took her in. She died young, while Coco lived on to a ripe old age.

In my late twenties there was "Jacob," the first dog of my first marriage. Jacob was a Lab-German Shepherd mix who was bought from a hippie commune outside of Ithaca, New York, where I was in graduate school at Cornell University, and prior to coming to our tiny A-frame home, had lived with his mother and his siblings under the front porch of the commune's farm house and had never been indoors. Jacob was a country dog for his first couple of years who ran in the woods every day with his local canine buddies, doing who knows what every day while we were at school or work. Over the years, he survived being hit by a car and shot in the rump by persons unknown and died from premature old age in Omaha, Nebraska, when my son Josh was a baby in 1977. After several years without a dog there came the saintly "Abby," another yellow Lab mix who was the dog of child-hood for my two children, Josh and Joanna. She was mostly left out of my life when Josh and Joanna's mother and I divorced (and I had only occasional visiting rights with Abby). Abby died peacefully in my arms at the end of her long life – more about that later.

The first dog of my second marriage was "Mac." He was a pure bred Yellow Lab. My wife Claire and I were planning to go out of the country for a year when he was 4 years old, and anticipating that long separation, I precipitously and ill-advisedly sent him away to live with our regular dog sitter (a vet herself), at a bad time between Claire and me. Looking back on it, I see this as an arrogant, selfish, and unthinking act for which I feel guilty always, and will do penance as long as I live. It took years for our relationship to recover enough to bring a new dog into our home. That dog was Dharma.

Dharma came to us in 2004. I found him – and he me – at the local SPCA when he was 3 months old. Claire and I had been vaguely looking for a new dog intermit-tently, for some time, but it took only minutes to decide on him – and apparently he on us. He is a quirky and intelligent canine – and while I love him dearly and he reciprocates, he is first and foremost Claire's "dog soul mate," as she refers to him.

The strength of their attachment and the intimacy of their communication are rare, even among those who greatly love their dogs. She often greets him in the morning with "I love you more today than I did yesterday." It is a struggle to find words capable of conveying the depth of her feelings for him. Perhaps coming closest is what dog behaviorist Patricia McConnell writes of her beloved departed dog Luke in her book "For the Love of a Dog": "And I still love him so deeply and completely that I imagine his death to be as if all the oxygen in the air disap-peared, and I was left to try to survive without it." (p. 4) [1] For Claire and Dharma it's like that, and when he became mysteriously ill in the Spring of 2009, and appeared to be in grave danger I thought Claire would herself give up the ghost if

Dharma did so. Dharma's X-rays, MRI, and CAT Scan never discovered definitively what was wrong, but fortunately for us all, he recovered through the intervention of veterinarians, acupuncturists, a sacro-cranial therapist, and a couple of animal communicators. Dharma got better and Claire survived.

Hope is a different sort of being. We found her – and she us – in 2007 at a crowded private shelter – called "New Hope," and run by a dedicated woman who was using her own salary to keep the place barely afloat. We went looking for a small fluffy white dog we had seen on the shelter's website, but were won over by the 1-year-old Black Lab-Beagle mix who had been rescued from a crack house where she had been abused and neglected for the first 6 months of her life (according to the shelter's report, "the man who had her hated her and used her as a punching bag.") Though the shelter called her "Midnight" in recognition of her profoundly black coat, we renamed her "Hope," in honor of the shelter that had rescued her from her tormentor.

She has certainly lived up to her name. Hope seems to wake up every day ready to appreciate her good fortune in life and to expect the new day will bring good things. If there is a canine positive psychology, then Hope is a proponent in her resilience, her joy, her life of commitment, and her dedication to being alive despite early deprivation, risk, and abuse.

If Dharma is Claire's dog, then Hope is mine. She is always ready for a tummy rub and cries pitifully when I leave the house (so I am told). She snores as loudly as I do some nights. My love for her is deep, and it is helping me to open my heart more fully to the joys of ordinary human life; she is my teacher in many ways.

If Dharma is an aristocrat – with fine features, long elegant legs, discerning tastes, a rare intelligence, and funny, quirky preferences – Hope is a plebian (and a drama queen), always ready to dive into smells in the woods and engage the world head on. I have learned much from both of them. Our morning walks are a chance to get a glimpse of the world through canine eyes (and noses). Knowing they need these three miles of walking and running each day helps me with will power to do myself the favor – even on cold and rainy days when staying home would be easier. They are good for my aging body, recently compromised by cardiac problems. But, more importantly, they are good for my soul.

Walking them provides a good time and place to think and contemplate, and to do so with their constant presence to focus and center me in what the Zen Buddhist teacher Thich Nhat Hanh calls "the present moment." And, they nurture in me all the traits I struggle to cultivate in my life: patience, selflessness, emotional responsiveness and expressiveness, and soulfulness. Truth be told, they do yeoman's work in making me a better person, if for no reason than I don't want to disappoint them or disprove the trust in me that they show each day through eyes and tail. Through them I align myself with the old saying "My goal is to be the person my dog thinks I am."

One of the tenets of humanistic and positive psychology is that we humans are not fixed and rigidly limited in what we can learn, how we can develop, and which behavioral habits we will cultivate. And neither are dogs, and our relationships with them (and perhaps with other animals) can shed important light on the possibilities of human potential.

Seligman's book *Authentic Happiness* [2] offers many pathways to the good life, including the fact that modern psychological research shows that the kind of positive mood associated with walking dogs in the park actually boosts human performance, expands the solutions that people generate in problem-solving, and enhances immune system functioning. Walking with Hope and Dharma certainly heightens my awareness, and as Daniel Gilbert [3] has demonstrated in his book *Stumbling on Happiness*, the capacity to be aware, to have imagination and to envision the future is precisely the defining characteristic of being human.

Awareness is the first step in human progress. Of course, to believe this requires belief in the reality of consciousness itself – no small matter in our world in which there is a tendency to reduce all mental activity to a matter of biochemical reactions, as if this explained all of experience. The Buddhist scientist Matthieu Ricard [4] (who became a monk after leaving a promising career in biochemistry) is among a growing number of scientists who recognize the reality of consciousness beyond biochemistry, and sees in it the key to the happiness we seek. Neuroscientist Mario Bureaugard [5] – the author of *The Spiritual Brain* – is another.

In a conversation with the French rationalist–humanist philosopher Jean-Francois Revel (who is his father) Ricard recounts the following example from Tibet about the transformational experience that led a man to become a Buddhist teacher (Lama): "There was also a lama just before the turn of the century who had lived, until he was 30, as a hunter and bandit (in Tibet, hunters are viewed with no less disapproval than bandits). One day, he was trailing a doe that he'd shot and mortally wounded. He caught up with the animal and found her collapsed on the ground. She lay there, bleeding and exhausted, and the hunter realized that she'd been giving birth. And he saw that, to her very last breath, her only concern was the newborn fawn she was lovingly licking. The sight completely overwhelmed the hunter, and he decided there and then to give up hunting. Soon the preoccupations of ordinary life began to seem futile and deceptive to him, and he devoted himself from then on to meditating on love and compassion and studying the scriptures. He became a famous teacher" [6] (in "The Monk and the Philosopher" pp. 58–59).

This is a message of hope because it links humanity to the various other beings that co-inhabit the planet with us in a relationship of spiritual equality. Just as the movement for "the rights of children" is a natural outgrowth of progress on the "rights of women" as females are permitted and encouraged to give voice to their experience, so the "rights of animals" follows naturally from an expanded appreciation for human rights as men, women, and children give voice to their experience and point in the direction of recognizing the "rights" of all sentient beings. It is indeed a moral circle of care that expands as consciousness evolves. I think that in this expanding consciousness lies the hope of the world. It is the foundation for our salvation as individuals and as a species on planet Earth. As we shall see, it is also at the heart of positive psychology.

Some scholars have speculated that the course of human evolution has produced in us a predisposition to be attuned to animals, to love other living beings – what is called the "biophilia hypothesis (a term popularized by the humanistic psychologist Erick Fromm [7]." In the current era, we face the challenge of halting and reversing the destructive effects of human-created climate change and environmental degradation, and one of the important criteria for evaluating the long-term success of positive psychology will be its contribution to this effort. As I was finishing this book, our collective consciousness was seared by the images of oil gushing from a broken well in the Gulf of Mexico and overwhelmed by the Brown Pelicans who were drowning in that oil. Biophilia is certainly one of the pillars for any position of hope in this world we face.

Now, and in the decades to come, caring for the Earth and its creatures (including ourselves) is the paramount political challenge before us as a species. Fulfilling the moral imperatives of our attunement to animals is essential to all of our relationships so that we may save the planet and therefore ourselves; we need the biophilia hypothesis now more than ever before. For me, and I believe for many others (some of whom do not even know it yet), our relationships with dogs provide perhaps an excellent opportunity – perhaps the best opportunity – to learn what we need to know to save the future of the planet as a whole and of ourselves as individuals.

Research conducted by Friederike Range et al. [8] in Austria provides a fascinating example of how the instinctive morality of dogs can provide instructive role models for humans. The researchers asked 43 dogs to extend their paws to humans (all of the dogs had learned this behavior prior to the experiment). After they established that all the dogs would perform the task (either alone or in the company of another dog), they introduced a reward into the situation. Specifically, they created situations in which two dogs were present. They then rewarded one dog for giving its paw to the researcher but did not reward the other dog. The result? Among the unrewarded dogs (who had observed the injustice of seeing the other dog rewarded for the same behavior that they exhibited), the rate of offering their paw when asked declined from 100 to 30% (13 of 43).

The researchers reported that the unrewarded dogs also showed more stress – as evidenced by licking or scratching themselves. It's not clear why the 13 dogs continued to offer their paw after observing injustice. Excessively hopeful? Unobservant? Particularly compliant? Perhaps future research will illuminate that point, but for now the study leaves the core message that dogs can and do respond to unfair treatment, and most experts believe this "value" of fairness is an evolutionary product – i.e., the ability to detect unfairness has survival value, and thus the norm of sharing is "natural" for social animals such as canines.

What can we conclude from this study? I believe it is that fairness (justice?) is a virtue to which dogs are sensitive. As the lead researcher reported, "They are clearly unhappy with the unfair situation." Paul Morris [9], a British animal behavior researcher, speculates that this is why dogs dislike seeing their owners being affectionate to other dogs (or even babies new to the family). We see this clearly with Hope and Dharma. I believe that they have a well-developed sense of fairness that operates in several ways. For one thing, they show the expectation that affection for one requires affection for the other. This expectation of equity is simply met when it comes to petting, if my wife and I are both present, and "tag team" petting is possible.

When one of us is alone with the two dogs, however, there is often a struggle for each dog to get his or her fair share of the affection being handed out by the beloved human.

Perhaps because she is younger, smaller, and newer to the family, Hope even has a special facial expression when she is struggling to get her fair share and express her anxiety that she is losing out. We call it "the teeth," because she raises her upper lip to show her top set of teeth. This is not a snarl, but a rather comical look that we only see otherwise on television or in movies when the image of a dog is digitally manipulated to produce a goofy smile. The first time we saw it in Hope, however, we were taken aback, but now we understand the message (and sometimes even evoke it by asking her to "show us the teeth"). Knowing this we try to maintain a scrupulous fairness in our dealings with Hope and Dharma.

When it comes to food, Hope and Dharma display confidence that the norm of sharing will be maintained. For example, they both love cheese. When there is cheese to be had they wait patiently, confident that a piece of cheese for one (usually Dharma first, as senior dog) will be followed with a piece for the other (usually Hope, waiting under the table while Dharma sits sentinel). It's a heart-warming demonstration of how much they trust us.

Dogs can enhance the natural impetus for fairness that is buried in the human genome. "Natural impetus for fairness"? Indeed, the concept of fairness is natural to human beings. This is not just the hypothesis of humanistic and positive psychology, it is the conclusion of evolutionary biologists and evolutionary psychologists who have studied this question empirically. Two who see the evolutionary impetus to fairness are Edmund O. Wilson [10] and Marc Hauser [1]. In his book *Moral Minds*, Hauser reviews research documenting that human beings – like dogs – come equipped with the capacity, indeed the inclination, to appreciate and value fairness. As such, it is part of a larger pattern that provides the foundation for my belief that living with dogs can stimulate moral development. Sometimes this moral inspiration lasts a lifetime.

A study of animal rights advocates reveals that most of them identified their childhood experiences *with* animals – particularly dogs – as the origins of their life's work *on behalf of* animals. Dog expert Patricia McConnell [1] is one who acknowledges this. In her book *For the Love of A Dog*, she writes "One of my earliest childhood memories is of lying on the living room floor wondering what was going on in the mind of my dog, Fudge. I wanted to know what she was thinking, what she was feeling. Even at the age of five or six I wondered, what is life like inside her soft, furry little head? Is she happy? Is she sad?" (p. 5). And those questions became the focal point of McConnell's adult life.

World famous naturalist Jane Goodall [11] is another. Although known for her appreciation for and advocacy on behalf of apes, she traces her professional life as an animal advocate to her childhood relationship with a dog. She writes "At age ten I developed a very special relationship with an extraordinarily intelligent mixed breed dog, Rusty, who became my constant companion. He, along with the three successive cats, two guinea pigs, one golden hamster, one canary, and two tortoises with whom we shared our house and our hearts, taught me that animals, at least those with reasonably complex brains, have vivid and distinct personalities, minds capable of some kind of rational thought, and above all, feelings." (p. xi).

These relationships, particularly the special bond with her dog, gave her a foundation to resist the simplistic and falsely mechanical view of animals her science teachers tried to impose on her. She says of this mechanistic view, "But I could not accept this – it absolutely contradicted all I had learned during my years with Rusty…" (p. xii). Similarly, ethologist Marc Bekoff [12], in his book *The Emotional Lives of Animals*, finds himself wondering how supposed scientists can hold to obviously false ideas of who dogs are and what they are capable of by asking, "Didn't they ever have a dog?" And he writes, "To live with a dog is to know first-hand that animals have feelings. It is a no brainer" (p. xx). And he goes still further to recognize that the beginning of an appreciation for the morality of how animals are mistreated by researchers and factory farms is to ask, "Would you do that to your dog?" (p. xxi). Indeed, Berkoff's comment is right on the mark in terms of moral development, because it highlights the fact that one of the keys to a positive psychology is understanding the imperatives to moral development, and this means creating a "circle of caring," a circle the having of which, research shows, contributes to enduring authentic happiness in one's life.

Within the circle of caring our moral "values" apply; outside it there are only rational calculations of interest and efficiency. Each of us has a circle of caring. I recall a billboard near a highway in Toronto that an animal rights group had installed to raise public consciousness about fishing. It featured a picture of a Yellow Lab and the question, "Why don't we fish for dogs?" Why indeed. Most of us would consider fishing for dogs to be immoral precisely because we include dogs in our circle of caring, whereas fish are outside the circle. There are many reasons for this, of course – our conceptions of the ability of dogs vs. fish to feel pain, for example.

As an aside, it is worth noting that even fish do feel pain according to modern research on the topic [13]. If taken into moral consideration, this finding should challenge the average fisher who has long justified the hooking and torture of fish on the supposition that these beings are without the capacity to feel pain. Even fish should be inside our circle of caring. And if fish, who else?

As Berkoff's comments suggest, however, not even all dogs are inside the typical human's circle of caring, and having dogs inside does not guarantee that all humans are as well. Adolph Hitler apparently loved his own dog – and he promoted strong animal welfare and protection laws at the same time he was advocating and implementing the extermination of millions of human beings. Many people who do have "pet" dogs seem indifferent to the suffering of other dogs with whom they do not have a personal connection (and who are thus outside the circle of caring).

But nonetheless, I think it is true that one of the important ways that dogs can be moral teachers is by moving us from an egocentric focus on self-interest to a broader focus on the welfare of others – other "sentient beings" as Buddhist teachers are prone to call them – including the nonhuman. This teaching seems clear in the lives of animal advocates – who, of course, may have been predisposed to an ethic of caring by reason of their temperament and parental role models. And it seems clear in Christian teachings that emphasize our moral responsibility to care for all other beings on the planet as part of our God-given mission to have "dominion" over animals, in the sense of taking responsibility to care for them (the good shepherd rather than the callous exploiter).

Moving beyond the ranks of professional researchers and advocates, many adults seem to have learned from the dogs of childhood positive lessons that they hold onto over the years, knowing that coming back to an animal-oriented life will be essential for them to feel they have completed their *human* purpose on Earth. At 53, my sister Karen is an example of this. She writes:

"I am the youngest in my family and the only girl. When I was seven, my parents let me pick out a puppy from a litter at a friend of ours house. A chubby brown and white puppy and I mutually chose each other, and I named her Coco. I was a chubby kid and had a cleft lip repaired, which when combined with my painfully shy nature, left me with few friends. Coco became the best friend I needed. She and I formed a bond that saw me through my early adolescence. While my love of animals has been with me since birth, Coco cemented that love. I now have three dogs and two horses and could no more imagine a life without my canine and equine family than I could without air or water. After I retire from my job in state government in a few years, I know that I will pursue a second career working with animals."

The status that dependent humans have in families and indeed in the entire society mirrors the status of dogs in the human community and can be an important basis for understanding important issues of moral development. How and where dogs (and other companion animals) lie within the human circle of caring can explain a great deal about how dependent beings generally are treated, and what lessons we can learn from that treatment. One way in which these lessons are taught is through the books and films that we read, see, and listen to.

Amazon.com lists more than 10,000 books of fiction that deal with dogs (vs. 6,000 that deal with cats). We can add to this the many volumes of what might be called "dog memoirs" – adults writing about their relationship with a particular dog (like *Merle's Door* [14] and *Marley and Me* [15]). These books – and the fictional accounts that outnumber them – provide adults and children with some of the cultural and psychological models for relationships with dogs, and in so doing, they often teach us how to be better human beings.

Consider as an example the classic story "Lassie." From the start, books of this sort have been seen as teachers – to wit this review by Lauren Peterson [16] (writing in *Booklist*): "*Lassie Come Home* – Eric Knight's 1938 classic about the loyal collie who refuses to accept her fate when she is sold, out of financial necessity, to a wealthy duke… Raising such issues as poverty, black lung disease, and cruelty to animals, this powerful story is a perfect tool for promoting empathy and compassion in youngsters."

Does it work, this "perfect tool"? It's hard to draw a straight causal line from books to behavior in children, but in the case of "Lassie," there is a bit of empirical research that sheds some light on this. A study conducted in the 1970s [17] examined the prosocial behavior of first graders who watched an episode of the "Lassie" TV show in which the main character – a boy named Jeff – rescues one of Lassie's puppies. These children were a bit more likely to help a real puppy when given the chance than children who watched a "neutral" (as opposed to "prosocial") TV program – but less likely to do so than similar children who experienced a role playing training program that explicitly focused on concepts and behaviors linked to empathy.

This study is consistent with many others showing that the effects of messages on TV are not as strong as messages that are "taught" more explicitly and with a simultaneous presentation of prosocial ideas ("cognitive structuring") and behaviors ("behavioral rehearsal"). Here we see the importance of context. The impact of literary messages about caring for dogs depends in part on how relevant those messages are to the children receiving them. Children who are living with dogs are best able to make good use of those messages. Developmental psychologist Lev Vygotsky [18] speaks of the importance of "scaffolding" in development, by which he means building incrementally upon experiences and ideas to reach higher levels. The literary treatment of dogs in the lives of children can be just such a process of scaffolding.

One of the most unaddressed but important topics for that scaffolding is the treatment of dogs in institutions across America. Nearly 100,000 dogs per year are used in medical research and some five million are killed at "shelters" that cannot place them or afford to maintain them [19]. These ugly facts are often hidden from most of us, but what lessons does this teach about life? Finding ways to educate ourselves about the dark side of life for dogs (as well as children with disabilities, the poor, the sick, and oppressed) in our society without traumatizing ourselves as learners is a big challenge, but one that we must take up. The fledgling "no kill" shelter movement is a natural base for educating humans about dogs, and what it means to include them in our circles of caring.

In November 2008, on the night of his election to the US Presidency, Barak Obama delighted the election-night crowd by affirming that his daughters would indeed be receiving a new puppy upon their arrival in the White House to take up residence as America's "First Family." No sooner were the words out of his mouth than nominations for this First Dog began arriving via the internet, facilitated by the mass media. One of the compelling dimensions of this dialog concerned the origins of the puppy, most notably if it would come from a shelter or from a breeder.

The case for adopting a shelter pup as a matter of public education is compelling. Best estimates are that dogs live in some 50 million American families [19]. Some 14% of them come from shelters (with 38% from pet stores or breeders and 48% from friends or by rescuing strays). At present, some five million dogs a year are killed in shelters because no one will adopt them. Estimates are that if the rate at which American families adopt shelter dogs (14%) were to double – to 28% – it would not be necessary to kill any shelter dogs, and all shelters could become "no kill shelters."

This is why advocates immediately saw the Obama family pup as an opportunity to send a message promoting the adoption of shelter dogs (as would a high-profile adoption of an American child in foster care send the same awareness-building message about children). When the Obama family chose a pure bred puppy – ostensibly because of allergy issues in the Obama children – shelter advocates felt the loss of an important teaching moment (and Vice-President Biden attempted to limit the damage by adopting a second dog to add to his family's pure bred pooch). Oh! How many teaching moments there are in the lives of dogs in relation to us humans – and how many are squandered.

However, the fact is that their relationship with human beings has not protected dogs from being exposed to cruelty, any more than their special place in our morality has protected children from parental and institutional maltreatment. Some of this cruelty is rooted in abnormal personality development in human beings: pathological individuals who manifest their disturbed thinking and feeling in the abuse of dogs. Cruelty to animals is often an important dimension of disturbed personality development in children, and often reflects troubled, even abusive family relationships [20].

Knowing how to recognize and deal with this is an important issue for anyone who cares about children and dogs (and other animals). Cruelty to animals is observed in some 25% of children who are diagnosed with Conduct Disorder [21] (a general pattern of aggression, bad behavior, and violating the rights of others that when it is observed in 10 years old, is about a third of the time the precursor to serious violent delinquency in adolescence). Often it is the first observable sign of this developmental problem that affects up to 10% of children in our society.

But some of the cruelty dogs experience is rooted in the cultural conception of dogs that informs the way we humans treat them. Cruelty abounds when dogs are seen as grossly inferior to human beings – as unfeeling and unthinking organisms. For example, the famous seventeenth century French philosopher Decartes is best known for his statement "I think therefore I am." But less well known is the fact that he rationalized hideous cruelty to animals on the grounds that they were "automata," not sentient beings, and thus could not feel pain, only exhibit mechanical behaviors in response to stimuli, mechanical behaviors that he repeatedly demonstrated [22].

To "prove" this, he and his followers nailed living dogs to barn doors and dissected them – until they died. In what was clearly extraordinarily callous and insensitive, Decartes maintained that the dogs' behavior (screaming and writhing) was not suffering at all – indeed did not indicate genuine feeling of any kind – but was merely mechanical reaction. It appears that he did not derive pleasure from this (and thus should not be considered a sadist, strictly speaking) except to the extent that he took pleasure in proving his point (and thus his sadism was mostly narcissistic and "theoretical"). I suppose the best that we could say of him is that he was emotionally stunted and spiritually shut down.

Can one ever take seriously the "philosophy" of such an individual after learning of this? I cannot, and no manner of "contextualizing" his behavior is likely to change my mind on that score. Scratch Descartes off my list of "philosophers worth taking seriously." Of course, his lack of compassion reeks of an extreme form of masculine emotional obliviousness as well as the position that the human species is the only one that counts morally and philosophically ("speciesism").

Beyond the psychologically troubled child who hurts dogs and the emotional coldness of macho mentality is the larger social problem of institutionalized cruelty, for example, dog fighting. This issue received a brief moment of public attention in 2007, with the revelation that a popular professional football player – Michael Vick – was involved in a dog fighting ring. Children and youth are often witnesses or even accomplices to this nastiness. Helping them come back from the dark side is often a matter of getting them to bring dogs into the circle of caring, and thus harnessing whatever caring impulses they may have.

I thought of this in 1997, when interviewing a violent delinquent boy named Malcolm [23], a boy who had admitted to several shootings, at least one of them fatal.

I knew from our earliest conversations that before he was arrested he was involved in a dog fighting ring that operated underground in his neighborhood. Over the months that I interviewed Malcolm, perhaps offering him the first genuinely caring relationship of his life, his moral calculus began to change concerning the pit bulls he used in the dogfights he had staged for profit. When we started our conversations, there were very clear boundaries about which dogs were inside and which were outside his circle of caring. He didn't use all his dogs in fighting, only those he had included in his world of expediency. He held back the few that were his "pets," including them in his circle of caring.

The change was this: after five months of our conversations Malcolm volunteered the information that he had decided he could no longer put *any* of his dogs in the ring and was giving them up. He had opened up to the emotional meaning of his actions regarding all the dogs. That is one of the keys to dogs as moral teachers, of course: once you open your heart you can see reality in a new way, you can see how there is nothing more important to feeding your soul a healthy moral diet than expanding your circle of caring as broadly as you can. Perhaps Michael Vick was touched this way. When he emerged from prison in 2009 he signed on to be an advocate against dog fighting with the American Humane Society's campaign to rid our society of this pernicious institution. Time will tell how genuine and durable that apparent change of heart turns out to be.

Beyond cruelty, there are other ways in which the relationships between humans and dogs are sometimes negative. Fear of dogs is quite common in young children – 69% of two year olds and 12% of four year olds according to one study [24] – but much less so in older children. Bad experiences with dogs often feed this fear. Over two million children are bitten by dogs each year in the USA – mostly dogs they know. Nearly 400,000 of these require treatment in an emergency room (and about a dozen children die from their injuries) [25]. These children quite possibly may continue being afraid or at least wary of dogs throughout their lives and be deprived of the important benefits of child–canine relationships. My wife Claire's story speaks of this possibility – and the alternative path that may be taken.

"I was 7 years old. Every day on my way to school I would walk by Ranger – our neighbors' German Shepherd. They kept him on a chain in their front yard that just barely reached the sidewalk. One rainy day as I walked by his house and strayed onto his lawn Ranger attacked me. He started growling and barking and then lunged at me. I don't know why this day was different, but something set him off. Before I could move he got my leg in his mouth and would not let me go. I screamed but no one heard me. Finally, I was able to crawl far enough where he could not reach me anymore. I still have the scars….and I am still afraid of German Shepherds. Luckily, I had my own dog at home – a small fuzzy one – that I could still connect with. As a result, I have been able to live with and love dogs despite what happened to me."

Of course anyone who has been bitten by a dog is naturally apprehensive. And, some dogs are very aggressive and are not worthy of trust (at least by strangers). Indeed, Hope and Dharma often bark at strangers and take time to become accustomed to new people, so I understand that the world of humans and dogs is not a simple matter. But Claire has found a way to take advantage of the positive possibilities of the human–canine bond; no one lives more closely with a dog than Claire does with Dharma and no one cares more about rescuing street dogs in the Third World countries we have visited. But what is also clear is her uneasiness when in the presence of a German Shepherd, encountered in the park or at the vet's office. To acknowledge her uneasiness toward German Shepherds does not invalidate the positive psychology of her transcending her fear, and so to be able to enter into a loving relationship with a canine.

The world is full of negatives, but it *can be* overflowing with positives nonetheless. This is one of Seligman's important messages about positive psychology. By choosing to live a life committed to virtues, human beings can be happier in their lives. By turning away from pessimism and negativity and toward optimism and positivity, we can experience greater authentic happiness. This is not merely an assertion on Seligman's part, it is grounded in modern psychological research [2].

The relationships that we can and do have with dogs (and other animals) are a vitally important aspect of our development as fully human beings. Our capacity to have these relationships and the nature of them tells us much about the imperatives of positive psychology. In these relationships we can learn much about the core goals of positive psychology, thriving, happiness, and fulfillment. There is much more to be done to harness the power of human–canine relationships as our understanding of both parties grows.

This includes an appreciation for the fact that many, if not most adults, leave childhood with unfinished emotional business – carrying with them into adulthood a wounded inner child – and that relationships with dogs in adulthood can serve as a bridge to this wounded inner child and play a role in healing, sometimes decades after moving past adolescence. I feel that very strongly in my relationship with Hope and Dharma. Anna Quindlen is an astute observer of this aspect of the human condition, as is evident in her book *Good Dog. Stay*, when she writes, "Human beings wind up having the relationships with dogs that they fool themselves they will have with other people. When we are very young, it is the perfect communion we honestly believe we will have with a lover; when we are older, it is the symbiosis we manage to fool ourselves we will always have with our children. Love unconditional, attention unwavering, companionship without question or criticism. I once saw a pillow that said I WOULD LIKE TO BE THE MAN MY DOG THINKS I AM. That about covers it. So the traits we ascribe to our dogs, the stories we tell ourselves about them are, at some level our own stories" [26].

This is but one way in which the spiritual needs of human beings can be met through the dogs with whom we share companionship in this life of ours. The potential of these relationships grows as our understanding of the scope of human and canine consciousness grows. At the end of the day, there are few things better in life than boys and girls walking with their dogs – no matter how old they are… the boys, the girls, and the dogs.

A dear friend of mine, child psychologist David Crenshaw, offers this account of how a dog can fill the gaps in a family plagued by emotional coldness and loss.

"In therapy, a 13-year-old boy, Keith, told me about the story of his dog named Onslo. Onslo was a mixed breed medium size dog who was in the family and

3 years old when Keith was born. Onslo was very friendly but he could on occasion be fiercely protective of his family. Onslo became a cherished companion for Keith. Onslo hung out in his room and often slept in his bed. Keith explained, 'He would never leave my side.' Onslo and his grandmother (who lived with the family) made up for an absence in Keith's life because he felt his parents never had time for him and they filled some of the void and relieved some of the loneliness he felt. Keith was brought to therapy after writing a poem called, 'I am the guy of pain' that was very alarming to his family and school. He was in such pain that suicidal risk was a great concern even though he denied active intent. A key precipitating factor in his acute depression and suffering was the sudden and unexpected death of his grandmother – 'the only person in my family who ever had time for me.' In the ensuing months, Onslo played a key role in providing continuing companionship and support to Keith. He said that Onslo had a way of telling when Keith was especially sad and in pain and would come around seeking Keith's attention that served to distract him from his pain and sadness. Recently, Onslo at the age of 16 also died but Keith is much stronger now and has been able to grieve fully the death of his life-long companion without falling back into acute depression."

Keith's relationship with the dog Onslo gave him hope and a reservoir of positive emotions that prepared him for loss, and protected him from depression. Research conducted by Seligman and his colleagues and published in the *American Psychologist* [27] demonstrates this point: involving people in experiences grounded in positive psychology results in less depression and more happiness. In this research, the two "happiness interventions" that produced the most enduring effects were "using signature strengths in a new way" (in which participants identified their particular strengths in life and then expanded their use of these strengths) and "three good things in my life" (in which the participants recorded three good things that happened each day and were guided to focus on the causes of these positive outcomes). I believe being involved with canine companions is an excellent way to stimulate and enhance happy interventions of this sort.

The special abilities of dogs (cats, horses, and other animals) to elicit positivity in humans are causing health care practitioners to recognize their potential value in new and important ways. Thousands of dogs are employed by professionals as "pet therapists" or as "assistants" to people experiencing mental and physical problems and disabilities. Psychoanalyst Boris Levinson pioneered in this approach with children through his dog Jingles. Stumbling serendipitously upon Jingles' ability to connect with and soothe troubled children, Levinson elaborated a strategy for dogs as "co-therapists" that was outlined in his 1997 book (with Gerald Mallon) *Pet-Oriented Child Psychotherapy* [28]. From all that we know about the sensitivity of dogs and their ability to communicate beyond adult language, it is hardly surprising that children whose emotional lives and communicative powers are stunted, blocked, or preoccupied with traumatic experiences should find canines to be excellent therapeutic partners.

Using dogs with children experiencing autism (which is an increasingly frequent problem for children, now thought to affect one in 100 children) has received especially high marks from parents, children, and professionals, as is evident in the following account offered by 39-year-old Bill.

"My son Tom is autistic. Try as we would, my wife and I could never get through to him, never connect emotionally at all. Then we got Ryder – a yellow lab puppy. Somehow Tom connected to Ryder in a way he never did with us. Two years later Tom is beginning to connect with us. All because of Ryder."

Beyond these clinical accounts and studies lies a whole range of dog healing that arises spontaneously and serendipitously. Fifty-two-year-old Brenda's account of her son's miraculous experience with a healing dog exemplifies this.

"When my son Jeff had just turned six he came down with Chicken Pox and for whatever reason suffered a serious stroke that left him with a slight impairment when he walked. The stroke also erased everything he had learned in preschool and kindergarten. I think the emotional trauma was harder on him than the physical trauma. Soon his schoolmates lost interest as he could not run and play with them. One morning a little black ball of fur was huddled in the bushes. You could not tell what it was except it was furry and underfed. Of course we took it in and named it Candy – and the little stinker immediately took over the house. This dog played with my son night and day, sat by his bedside (or rather hid under the covers) and brought that special sparkle back to my son's eyes. The doctors were astonished at the progress that was made, having largely given up on him already. A child they thought would need special services was suddenly transformed into a rambunctious and mischievous little boy who made the soccer team the following year. This little dog stayed in our lives for about 5 years. She ran out to meet my son's school bus one day and was hit by a car. The driver had dropped a cigarette and was not watching the road. The car swerved off the road and hit the dog. I am confident this dog was a gift from above. Without Candy my son would have given up. I feel 99% of healing comes from the mind. This dog helped him forget he was sick and gave him the strength and courage to be a little boy again. Every time I see a little black dog I think to myself 'Thanks Candy, I owe you one!' "

I believe that there is no doubt that our relationships with dogs can be healing – physically, emotionally, even spiritually. This should not be surprising given how long dogs and humans have lived with each other, changing to become a better match through cultural *and* biological evolution.

Dogs were the first domesticated animals. Archeological research demonstrates that dogs have lived side by side with human beings all over the planet for *at least* 10,000 years – in some places 15,000 years [29]. Genetic research demonstrates that wolves and dogs diverged biologically and split into different species about 100,000 years ago. If human beings played a role in the genetic history of dogs, this would push back the date for starting the relationship between humans and dogs many tens of thousands of years beyond current archeological evidence, and as we shall see, this would support an intriguing hypothesis about the role of dogs in the early success of our species on the planet.

Whenever this relationship began, what is clear is that no other animal has lived so intimately with us for such a long time, and been so intertwined with our lives as human beings. Ancient burial sites have revealed the skeletons of puppies buried with human children. Of course, no one knows exactly how the affiliation of dogs and human beings began, but what is clear that it began with the process by which wolves were drawn into the human orbit.

Whenever the process began, some have speculated that children played a crucial role. They imagine that some wolves – perhaps the most bold or needy – were drawn to the human community by the smell of roasting flesh over cooking fires. Children could have served as ambassadors, perhaps tossing a half eaten bone to a curious wolf. Because they would be less threatening to these wolves than adults, children might have succeeded in initiating contact where adults might have been less interested or capable. Perhaps in their playful wanderings around the camp children discovered abandoned wolf pups and adopted them, saying the words that untold millions of parents have heard ever since, "Can I keep him... please!" However it happened, what did happen was the start of something big, something that continues to the present day.

One of the intriguing speculations about the special character of the human–canine bond concerns the very triumph of our species over prehistoric rivals, most notably the Neanderthal [30]. Current archeological research suggests that the human beings (Homo Sapiens) and Neanderthals coexisted in parts of the Earth 30,000–45,000 years ago. The Neanderthal was the dominant population in the Eurasian region for nearly 200,000 years before Homo Sapiens began to move out of their evolutionary home in Africa. The meeting of the two species was not a harmonious and pleasant one, by all accounts.

When all was said and done – only several thousand years after the first contacts – Neanderthal disappeared and Homo Sapiens took over (and have been the dominant hominid ever since). Why didn't the Neanderthal triumph? They were physically tougher, stronger, and even had larger skulls (thus implying the possibility of larger brains). Researchers have offered numerous possible explanations for the success of Homo Sapiens against the obvious advantages held by Neanderthal. The most intriguing of all from my perspective is offered by Stanley Coren (in his book *The Modern Dog*) [29].

The archeological evidence (bones at living and burial sites) indicates that while Homo Sapiens lived with dogs, Neanderthals did not. If dogs lived with humans longer than the 15,000 years ago limit that the evidence documents and more like the 50,000 years or more than some archeologists believe, Coren could be correct in his belief that it was the fact that human beings faced Neanderthals with canine companions that tipped that balance.

Why? Coren supposes that dogs served as an early warning system – their barking could alert human communities of the approach of intruders. This would have allowed better defensive responses by human communities. It even would have allowed humans to sleep better (obviating the need for posting guards through the night). Neanderthals did not have this advantage. Also, as the weaponry for hunting changed to employ arrows, which led to many wounded animals, humans would have been better positioned to succeed because their dogs could track, chase, and corner wounded animals more effectively than either Homo Sapiens or Neanderthals alone. The cumulative effect of the advantages of having canine partners could have led to the gradual extinction of the Neanderthal.

This hypothesis is by no means proven, given the lack of archeological evidence that links humans to dogs at the exact times and places where Homo Sapiens and Neanderthals were in competition. However, if it is true, it means that we human beings may owe our very existence to the ancestors of today's dogs. What is indisputable, is that in modern times many soldiers owe their lives to dogs.

As Harris Done's 2009 documentary "War Dogs of the Pacific" [31] makes clear, in many contemporary combat situations dogs do give their human allies a significant advantage (of the sort that Coren supposes they gave humans in their conflicts with Neanderthals). Done documents how the hundreds of dogs trained to deploy in the battles for the Pacific islands in World War II (Guam, for example) provided an often life-saving advantage for American soldiers and marines as they fought their Japanese counterparts in thick jungle. The dogs used their exquisite sense of smell and hearing to detect enemies long before their human counterparts could. What is more, the presence of the dogs allowed soldiers to sleep soundly at night on the front lines without fear of their enemies sneaking up on them in the darkness. Pictures of Marines sleeping in their fox holes with dogs by their sides in Done's film evoke the images that Coren provided of homo sapiens sleeping without fear of Neanderthal attack at night many thousands of years ago.

Soldiers from the wars in Vietnam a generation ago and in Iraq more recently echo the soldiers of World War II in testifying to the life-giving service their scout dogs provided. Perhaps we should begin every human–canine encounter with a bow of thanks. This would certainly go a long way to dispelling the idea that it is only dogs who should be thankful to us for our benevolence!

In any case, in the centuries that followed the first inclusion of wolves in the human circle, dogs evolved in ways that maximized their readiness to be human companions (and their usefulness to the human enterprise). Today, while their genetic origins in the wolf population is indisputable, equally clear is their distinctive adaptation to be human companions, including their retention into adulthood of what in wolves are juvenile traits (e.g., attributes like barking, which is virtually nonexistent in adult wolves but was cultivated by early human breeders, to wit the story of how Homo Sapiens defeated Neanderthals). The specialized canine traits that make dogs such great companions for human beings includes their sensitivity to verbal and nonverbal communication, their emotional expressivity, and their capacity for bonding in social groups like families. I believe that it also includes a psychic capacity for intuitive communication and attunement with human beings.

The special evolutionary history of the human–dog bond testifies to the importance of understanding not just the actual but also the potential of the human–dog bond. Over centuries of evolution and selective breeding, dogs became "more" than wolves in many ways (as well as "less" than wolves in others). But this is not a static process confined to ancient history. Indeed most of the recognized breeds of dogs today are of relatively recent origins. One of the remarkable biological characteristics of dogs is the fact that they naturally replicate genetic changes much faster than most other beings. This means that they can evolve quicker than other animals, and it makes them particularly susceptible to human genetic engineering (in the traditional form of selective breeding as well as in new and future efforts to directly manipulate genetic material).

But this appreciation of the enormous biological possibilities of dogs is not the whole story. There is more. Beyond our understanding of their potential for becoming more and different biologically is their capacity for what can only be called their "psychological" development. They, like human beings, can develop beyond the constricted images some cultures and individuals profess. One of the core interests of positive psychology is an enhanced and expanded understanding of human potential, and understanding how the potential of dogs can and does grow beyond limited concepts that some people hold onto is exemplary in this process.

The potential of both humans and dogs to develop cognitively and emotionally has long been underestimated by observers who don't understand the crucial role of social context in creating the conditions for advanced development – be it among canines or human. It is certainly true that if human children are raised in families where there is little verbal interaction and cognitive stimulation they usually do not develop to be what they could be if exposed to other, more stimulating and interactive settings. Interestingly, the rising IQ scores of Americans over the past century are attributed to a general increase in the degree to which kids are exposed to this kind of interaction and stimulation – by parents and by the mass media [32]. Today's human beings are capable of more because they are exposed to more, and they grow into those new possibilities.

If you drew conclusions about the potentialities of human beings to throw, catch, and hit a ball without ever seeing a Major League baseball player you would indeed have an impoverished conception of human potential in this domain. And, if you were unfamiliar with the Zen Buddhist teacher Thich Nhat Hanh's meditative capacity you might not believe that someone could have dental work done without anesthesia and feel no pain. Likewise, until you have heard Yo Yo Ma play the cello or witnessed the intellectual activity of a mathematical genius you could easily underestimate the human potential for music making and number crunching.

The same is true of dogs: they have greater potential than many humans recognize. Both human children and canine pups are capable of more competence than some of us realize precisely because we often deprive children and puppies of experiences to develop that competence. For example, some researchers have maintained that dogs have no sense of self, no ability to recognize their existence as a separate being (the way humans, elephants, dolphins, and chimps can). The evidence offered in support of this view is that when placed in front of a mirror in a laboratory situation, dogs show no indication that they realize the images in the mirror are themselves (the way children, elephants, and chimps do) 32.

Case closed? Not necessarily. In his book *Merle's Door*, naturalist Ted Kerasote [33] shows that his dog (Merle) was capable of understanding that the image in the mirror was himself. How and why? When Merle was alone in front of a mirror he indeed did not seem to register the self-identity of the image. However, when Ted and Merle were in view in a mirror side by side together – a social context that matches the essentially social nature of canine identity – the dog clearly processed the information. Here's Kerasote's lovely description of this event.

"Merle stopped dead and looked sharply up at me; then he looks back to the mirrored wall and gazed at my reflection. His mouth parted slightly and he cocked his head quizzically. I was obviously standing beside him, but I was also standing alongside that dog in the mirror.... Leaning forward, he gazed with intense concentration at the man and dog in the mirror and tentatively wagged his tail. The reflection of the dog wagged its. As if the rug had been pulled out from beneath him, Merle sat down. He turned his head up to me in wonder; he looked back to the mirror then he looked back to me. He began to wag his tail with considerable vigor. 'I get it,' his expression said. 'I see who I am.' The big mirror, taking in the entire room and all its occupants, had apparently let him see himself alongside people who he recognized from the real world. It had provided him with the necessary context to understand what a reflection was." (p. 232) Was Kerasote attributing understanding to Merle that he in fact did not have? After living with dogs as I have, I don't think so.

Positive psychology draws on one of the core principles of humanistic psychology, namely that our potential is usually greater than commonplace assumptions would have us think. If you create an impoverished environment for a human or a dog you will end up with a less intelligent being, be it human or canine than if you offer developmentally enhancing experiences.

One area where human (and canine) potential has long been underrated is the ability of the brain to change once it has matured in adulthood. For dogs this is captured in the old saw, "you can't teach an old dog new tricks." For humans, the message was expressed in the firmly held belief that adult human brains are not generally able to reconfigure to compensate for injuries or illnesses that impair functioning tied to specific areas of the brain. The new field of "neuroplasticity" says otherwise. This is captured in physician Norman Doidge's book *The Brain That Changes Itself* [34]. Doidge documents exciting new advances in the scientific study of the brain that show its amazing capacity to reconfigure in response to experience – for better or for worse. He describes the work of applied researchers ("neuroplasticians") who have found ways (often through creative technologies) to teach brains to do things that had been lost because of injury or illness – such as sight and balance. This provides the scientific foundation for studies showing that people who meditate consistently can retrain their brains – altering the pattern of use and energy.

And this is all the more true if you actively seek to increase the competence of both sets of beings through the way you interact with them. And this leads to a very big question indeed: *Are dogs enlightened?*

Of course, I know that from an everyday human perspective dogs can be quite "low," even disgusting. After all, they sometimes eat deer turds and think that rotting carcasses in the woods are a delight to roll in. And they seem powerless to avoid the temptation to chase squirrels. But then we human beings can be quite "low" and even disgusting ourselves. If you watch Chef Anthony Bourdain's television program "No Reservations" in which he travels the world in search of exotic culinary experiences, you know that humans eat some disgusting things too. Cheese curds covered in dirt and ashes? Hagus? Cotton candy? Insects? And we have a lot of compulsions ourselves, like pornography and reality TV. Does that make human beings exempt from the possibility of enlightenment? I don't think so.

Dogs can't do much math, can't read, can't speak human languages (but can understand words), and can't play or write music as human beings can. But then dogs can do a lot of things that humans can't do with their senses – like differentiate subtle smells and find their way home over long distances without maps or compasses (skills that some other animals demonstrate as well). Dogs don't have thumbs like we humans do, but they do have tails that wag.

Whatever limitations dogs have in comparison with human beings, I nonetheless think about their enlightenment often. I do so every time I encounter a dog who has an "objective" physical disability but who does not appear to be caught up in self-pity. Many mornings when Hope and Dharma and I walk in the park we encounter a young woman and her dog companion – Connie. There is nothing remarkable about the woman – except perhaps her constant simple smile – but the dog is unusual in having only three legs (his left front leg having been amputated). Why does this inspire thoughts of enlightenment?

It does so because it seems to exemplify one Buddhist definition of enlightenment – "to accept reality exactly as it is in every moment." The three-legged dog shows no sense of self-pity because of his disability. Of course, there are those who would argue that this simply demonstrates that dogs lack self-awareness entirely, as we shall see shortly.

The three-legged dog simply acts fully within his physical reality. This is an important way in which the acceptance contained within the definition of reality differs from "resignation." Resignation implies a chronic mourning for loss – perhaps a sad acceptance of reality coupled with longing. That longing is what is absent from the three-legged dog's acceptance. He is fully what he is – apparently not besieged by regrets for what might have been or jealousy when he sees what other dogs have, namely four legs. He is what positive psychology strives to understand and humanistic psychology strives to promote in human beings, a self-actualized individual whose experience is not defined by what they lack but rather by what they are, a glass always half full and never half empty.

This means a lot to me as I come to terms with my own limitations, as an aging man with a serious heart problem. I struggle with the loss of vitality each day as we repeat the walk Hope and Dharma and I have made for years now. I am reminded each day that I cannot walk as fast as I could only a few years ago. And I understand that an important measure of my spiritual development is my ability to achieve what the three-legged dog has accomplished, to demonstrate the same sense of *positive* acceptance with neither regret nor passive resignation. I felt this strongly when I went beyond my own first hand encounter with the three-legged dog to watch a couple of YouTube videos of *two*-legged dogs.

One – Dominic – lost both his right legs to amputation after an encounter with a car; the other – Faith – was born without her front legs. There is some sense to be made of focusing on the loss of the first dog. After all, he lived for a couple of years with four legs. His owner reports that after the surgery the dog simply jumped up and ran (on the two left legs remaining to him). Did it mean something to him? Did he sense the difference? Knowing dogs it is hard to imagine he was not aware of the *change*. And therein lies the spiritual point – to define and experience the transition from four to two legs as change rather than loss is the key. Every spiritual teacher – particularly those speaking from a Buddhist perspective – understands that experiencing change rather than loss – *or gain* – is the key to enlightenment: accepting reality exactly as it is in every moment.

And what of Faith, the two-legged dog who was born that way? Even to describe her that way is to miss the point. It is not that she is without "her two front legs," but that she was born with two legs (which in comparison with other dogs are "hind" as opposed to "front"). For her, they are not "hind" legs. *They are her legs.* She walks with the legs she has. She lives in the present moment. She accepts reality exactly as it is, as does Dominic. Good dogs. I aspire to be so enlightened; I work at it. I recall that in the mornings when Dharma and Hope and I meet the three-legged dog, when my leg is aching and my heart is tired. Good dogs.

But are dogs really enlightened? There is a classic Zen Buddhist text that speaks to this. It begins in the form of a traditional "koan" (a puzzling anecdote or riddle which has no objective answer, but which, like a parable, serves a teaching function) concerning a great Zen teacher of the late eighth and early ninth centuries named Chao-chou. "A monk asked Chao-chou: 'Does a dog have a Buddha-nature or not?' Chao-chou replied: 'He does not.'" According to Buddhism scholar T. Griffith Foulk [35], this simple negative answer is deceiving. As Griffith explains, all sentient beings have a Buddha-nature, but "unless they realize that fact by 'seeing the nature,' they remain caught up in delusion and continue to suffer in the karmically condition round of rebirth."

This is not the place to get into a long discussion of karma and rebirth (two Buddhist concepts that I struggle with, admittedly). Suffice it to say that the issue of awareness is central to Buddhist thinking about enlightenment, and I shall return to it later (in the next chapter). Here I will just say that dogs appear to generally do a better job of "accepting reality exactly as it is in every moment" than most people do (thus getting them at least on the road to enlightenment) even if they are not particularly good at self conscious self-awareness.

Daniel Gilbert's *Stumbling on Happiness* [3] is clear on this point: animals lack the brain to engage in the kind of imagination required of self-awareness and thus ultimately, enlightenment. But when it comes to the Dharma and Hope, I am not sure that they would see the point in that, not when there are bones to be had, balls to chew, squirrels to chase, and treats to be negotiated from their human companions.

Having said all this, I still maintain that walking with dogs can be a wonderful workshop in positive psychology. It reminds me always of what potential means, what happiness is, what fulfillment looks like, what thriving feels like. Seeing them I learn important lessons about all of Martin Seligman's three important dimensions. I learn about the life of fulfillment; walking with them is the simplest pleasure of life and demonstrates for me the satisfaction of ordinary living. I learn about the "life of engagement" because as I fulfill their need for a morning time in the woods I feel the beneficial results that come from giving your all to some activity and I feel the "flow." And, I understand better than I have ever before the "life of affiliation" as I experience the sense of worthwhileness that comes from contributing to things beyond myself. Dharma and Hope show me all this each morning, in each walk filled with present moments of joy and contentment and wonder. It's a good start. But this is not a book about dogs – although the dogs are always present in my mind (and often in the room) when I write. This is a book about being human, being human in time and place, about the human potential for being positive.

References

1. McConnell, P. (2007) For the love of a dog. New York: Ballantine Books.
2. Seligman, M. (2004) Authentic happiness. New York: Free Press.
3. Gilbert, D. (2007) Stumbling on happiness. New York: Vintage.
4. Ricard, M. and Goleman, D. (2007) Happiness: A guide to developing life's most important skill. Boston, MA: Little, Brown.
5. Bureaugard, M. and O'leary, D. (2008) The spiritual brain: A neuroscientist's case for the existence of the soul. New York: HarperOne.
6. Ricard, J., Ricard, M., Conti, J. and Miles, J. (2001) The monk and the philosopher: A father and son discuss the meaning of life. New York: Shocken, pp. 58–59.
7. Fromm, E. (1989) The art of living. New York: Peter Lang Publishers.
8. Range, F., Horn, L., Viranyi, Z. and Huber, L. (2009) The absence of reward induces inequality aversion in dogs. Proceedings of the National Academy of Sciences of the United States of America. 106(1), 340–345.
9. Morris, P. http://dsc.discovery.com/news/2006/08/23/jealousdog_ani.html.
10. Hauser, M. (2007) Moral minds. New York: Harper Perennial.
11. Goodall, J. (2007) Forword in Berkoff, M. The emotional lives of animals. Novato, CA: New World Library. p. xi.
12. Bekoff, M. (2008) The emotional life of animals. New York: The New American Library.
13. Chandroo, J. P., Duncan, I. J. and Moccia, R. D. (2004) Can fish suffer? Perspectives on sentience, pain, fear and stress. Applied Animal Behaviour Science. 86, 225–250.
14. Kerasote, T. (2008) Merle's door. New York: Harvest Books.
15. Grogan. J. (2008) Marley and me. New York: Harper.
16. Peterson, L. http://www.amazon.com/Lassie-Come-Home-Knights-Original-Classic/dp/0805064230/ref=sr_1_2?ie=UTF8&s=books&qid=1277738631&sr=1-2.
17. Sprafkin, J., Liebert, R. and Puolos, R. (1975) Effects of a prosocial televised example on children's helping. Journal of Experimental Child Psychology. 20, 119–126.
18. Vygotsky, L. and Kozulin, A. (1986) Thought and language. Cambridge, MA: MIT Press.
19. http://www.humanesociety.org/issues/pet_overpopulation/facts/overpopulation_estimates.htmlNumber of dogs in American homes.
20. Ascione, F. and Arkow, P. (1999) Child abuse, domestic violence, and animal abuse: Linking the circles of compassion for prevention and intervention. West Lafayette, IN: Purdue University Press.
21. Gleyzer, R., Felthous, A. and Holzer, C. (2002) Animal cruelty and psychiatric disorders. Journal of American Academy of Psychiatry and Law. 30, 257–265.
22. Donovan, J. (2007) Animal rights and feminist theory. In J. Donovan and C. Adams (Eds.) The feminist care tradition in animal ethics. New York: Columbia University Press, pp. 58–86.
23. Garbarino, J. (1999) Lost boys. New York: Free Press.
24. Rutter, M. (1987) Developmental psychiatry. Washington, DC: American Psychiatric Publishing.
25. http://www.dogbitelaw.com/.
26. Quindlon, A. (2007) Good dog, stay. New York: Random House.
27. Seligman, M., Steen, T., Park, N. and Peterson, C. (2005) Positive psychology progress. American Psychologist. 60, 410–421.
28. Levinson, B. and Mallon, G. (1997) Pet-oriented child psychotherapy. New York: Charles Thomas.
29. Coren, S. (2008) The modern dog. New York: Free Press.
30. Hall, S. (2008) Last of the Neanderthals. National Geographic, October.
31. http://www.uswardogs.org/.
32. http://www.pbs.org/newshour/forum/april98/iq_4-20.html.
33. Kerasote, T. (2007) Merle's door. New York: Harcourt.
34. Doidge, N. (2007) The brain that changes itself. New York: Penguin.
35. Foulk, T. G. http://www.beliefnet.com/Faiths/2000/07/Does-A-Dog-Have-Buddha-Nature.aspx. New York: Vintage.

Chapter 2
The Costs and Benefits of Obliviousness: Growing Up in the 1950s

I was born in 1947, so I spent most of my childhood in the 1950s (and thus my adolescence in the 1960s) as a member of what is commonly referred to as the "Baby Boomer" generation. The name comes from the fact that after the relatively low birth rate associated with the Great Depression of the 1930s and the disruption of World War II (when more than eight million served in the military forces), with the end of the War and the return of the troops and prosperity, there was an explosion of births. From 1945 to 1946, the number of babies born in the USA jumped from 2.8 to 3.5 million per year and peaked in 1957 with a figure of 4.3 million [1]. It then held relatively steady for years to come as the siblings of the first wave of Baby Boomers were born and joined the swollen ranks of their older brothers and sisters (my younger brother was born in 1951 and my sister in 1958).

The year I was born, the hospital in which my mother delivered in Manhattan was so crowded that her bed was in the hallway. By the time I started school, a building boom was underway to accommodate the escalating number of children showing up to be educated, and from then on I and my age-cohort were treated to a mixture of hastily erected temporary classrooms, new buildings, and split sessions (half the students started early in the morning and finished by lunch, while the other half started after lunch and finished in the late afternoon). This was to continue through elementary school, into junior high school and on into high school, only to be followed by similar experiences in college, when institutions scrambled to increase capacity and the number of campuses increased dramatically.

This demographic reality had a significant effect on the shape and texture of the second half of the twentieth century [2]. It had implications for the economy (rapid growth) and culture (Woodstock), as this market opportunity generated all kinds of enterprises that in the 1960s focused on youth-related activities, in the 1990s focused on adult vacations, second homes, efforts to improve middle-age sex, and as the twenty-first century moves forward a focus more and more on retirement-related matters (a good time to invest in the "Mick Jagger Retirement Home," where the issue will indeed be whether or not you "can't get no satisfaction").

But all that was in the future when I was a child, growing up in the 1950s. It is more than self-indulgence to reflect on childhood (and parenting) in the 1950s, however, because I believe it is a useful and important exercise, in part for what it

J. Garbarino, *The Positive Psychology of Personal Transformation:*
Leveraging Resilience for Life Change, DOI 10.1007/978-1-4419-7744-1_2,
© Springer Science+Business Media, LLC 2011

can tell us about the utility of positive psychology in attempts to understand human lives. After all, many people consider the 1950s to have been "the happy decade."

During the 1950s, I lived in what I thought to be an average family, in an average community. By the standards of the time, I thought we were middle class, despite the fact that neither of my parents had graduated from high school, and we went through some hard economic times when my father was unemployed. This belief that we were middle class nonetheless is not remarkable by virtue of the fact most Americans (then and now) consider themselves middle class. In a recent poll, about 90% of us identified ourselves as middle class in one way or another (with 2% saying that they were in the "upper class" and 7% saying that they were in "the lower class") [3]. Indeed, one of the economic triumphs of the post-World War II era was that "working class" families (with blue- and pink-color jobs) could aspire to and even realize what were traditionally the hallmarks of middle class life – for example, cars, vacations, and the possibility of sending their children to college.

When I was growing up we always had food on the table. Although I lived in a public housing project in the early 1950s, it was at a time when that was a privilege for aspiring and upwardly mobile families entering the middle class, and by 1956, we owned our own home. We had a car and a television set. We went to the movies from time to time. We went on vacation every few years (to visit relatives). But from a modern child's perspective, we might appear to have been poor. We didn't go out to eat more than twice a month. Our house had only one bathroom. We had only one car and one television set, and we bought clothes mainly each September at back-to-school sales. From the time I was 13 years old, I had a paper route to earn spending money, and we played ball on the street in front of our house.

My children belong to a different world, not just because of the fact that when they were little I made much more money than my father ever did while I was a kid. Having been born in the 1976 and 1982, respectively, as children my Josh and Joanna and my step-son Eric lived in a different world than I did because the social environment is very different from what it was in the 1950s. The world of my childhood is nearly unfathomable to them. They cannot really believe what my life was like as a kid growing up in the 1950s in the New York metropolitan area. They have difficulty understanding the nostalgic pride with which I talk about the relative simplicity of those times. TV had entered our lives, but with only four channels and no VCR or DVDs. When we played on the street it was in canvas sneakers, not leather running shoes. We had board games such as Monopoly and Scrabble, but no video games.

When we thought about the world, it was in simple, child-sized terms, not with the apparent sophistication of today's kids. The people across the street got furious if you accidentally hit a ball onto their lawn, but no one thought of suing anybody over it. The man down the street did some crazy things (like dressing up one New Year's Eve as the New Year's Baby, and then getting into a car accident in his car and getting arrested), but we did not know that he was an alcoholic. It was not until I was 20 years old that I understood the meaning of the fact that when I was 3 years, my mother and I had gone to live with her parents for the better part of a year (more on that later).

When they were young, I sometimes tried to explain to my children what life was like when I was a kid, and was left feeling a bit like a dinosaur trying to explain what life was like before mammals when I talked to them about the old days. They know about divorce first hand. They could not grow up without becoming aware of rape and murder and the other staples of the daily news: about AIDS, drugs, genocide, and sexual abuse. It was not until I was an adult professional that I realized with a bolt of clarity that the girl down the street *must* have been sexually abused and that the older brother of my friend up the street *must* have been gay. Neither "sexual abuse" nor "homosexual" was a concept with which many children of my era were familiar (unless perhaps they had first hand family or individual experience, and even then they may not have realized what they were experiencing in many cases).

One day in the late 1980s, my kids and I were driving in our car in Chicago, reenacting a routine many parents know well. My daughter was speaking for the realities of her times. I was trying to explain what was gone and what was missing, whatever benefits may have accrued in the changing times. I suppose I had assumed the instructional mode into which we parents often sink when making a point with our offspring. Finally, my daughter put all nostalgia in its place: "Dad," she said with a rhetorical flourish, "it ain't the 1950s anymore." Indeed it isn't.

It is not the core themes and concerns of childhood that differ from age to age and place to place. Rather, it is the cultural, psychological, and social messages and tools that children have available to them as they go about the universal business of growing up. The nature of these messages and tools can have an effect on that process of growing up, however. While many are merely shifts in cultural style, some are positive rather than negative. Some do ennoble; others do degrade. Some promote social order; others promote chaos. Some are good; some are bad.

Some result in young adults who want to serve humanity and carve out a spiritually meaningful life for themselves, like the kids I read about who raised money in their school to help Hurricane Katrina victims a thousand miles away. Others result in teenagers like the ones I watched on a "reality" program on television who to a person said their goal in life was "to be rich and famous."

A positive psychology of childhood seeks to understand how and why character and happiness and the capacity for joy flourish in some children and languish in others. There have always been both kinds of kids in America. The issue is whether there was something about the 1950s that affected the ratio between the positive and the negative in kids' lives, between the toxic and the nurturing, and thus the balance of positive power in the social environment.

Amidst all the confusion and the temptations and the blind alleys of modern life, we can always gain clarity by asking the positive question, "does this contribute to my character development?" In answering this question as in every other developmental issue, we must always remember that context matters, indeed often overwhelmingly so. Rarely does the process of cause and effect work universally in matters of human development. Rather, it operates in the context established by family as family itself operates within the context of neighborhoods and community, of socioeconomic systems, of culture, of gender and ethnicity, of prior experience, and of historical circumstance. This is the fundamental lesson we learn from scientific research on human development. When we look at the development of children and ask, "does x cause y?" the best scientific answer is almost always "it depends" [4].

It depends. That is one of the most important messages from modern developmental science, and it provides the foundation for an ecological perspective as laid out by my mentor, developmental psychologist Urie Bronfenbrenner beginning in the 1960s [5, 6]. Urie's books *Two Worlds of Childhood* (1970) and *The Ecology of Human Development* (1979) pioneered in making the case for the paramount importance of context in shaping the workings of developmental influences, influences that are found in the child's biology, the child's psychology, the child's family, the child's schools, the child's community, the child's society, and the child's culture.

A direct implication of this ecological perspective is the fact that rarely if ever does a single influence determine the course of a child's life, *for better or for worse.* Whether these influences be negative – "risk factors" – or positive – "developmental assets" – it is extremely rare that a single influence is decisive [7]. Rather, it is the accumulation of risk factors and the accumulation of developmental assets that generally describe the level of social toxicity and social robustness, which when coupled with the forces of human biology tell the story of a child's development.

Knowing this can help guide us as I proceed with my reminiscence of growing up in the 1950s because I want to find a path between nonreflective glorification and anachronistic criticism. As the talented novelist and editor Peter de Vries put it so well a generation ago, "Nostalgia just isn't what it used to be" [8]. Looking back on it, with today's informed eyes, I know life in the 1950s was neither a fully realized time nor a social utopia. Acknowledging that it was a glass neither full nor empty, was the glass half empty or half full?

The answer, I think is "yes, half full and half empty," but with a twist, one that Martin Seligman builds upon in his analysis of the roots of authentic happiness. His reading of the research tells him that the best way to look at the glass is the optimistic solution: to overestimate the positive and underestimate the negative *even if this is at odds with "objective" reality* [9]. The surest path to depression is the pessimist's approach – to do the opposite by underestimating the positive and overestimating the negative (*or even accurately assessing the negative!*). This, I think, is a key to the benefits of 1950s obliviousness: depression was at lower levels because the culture was optimistically underestimating the negatives and overestimating the positives! There is a bumper sticker that says, "If you're not outraged you're not paying attention!" True perhaps, but sadly true. Knowledge may be power, but ignorance can be bliss, and obliviousness very reassuring.

I want to see what was good and true about that era, as a way of recognizing in place some of the key elements of positive psychology. At the same time, I want to have a perspective that will allow me to identify and articulate the secret wrongs, the unspoken pain, and the lack of awareness that were as characteristic of the era as well as its simple benefits and pleasures. I want to use this reflection on growing up in the 1950s as an opportunity to consider the pros and cons of what I consider to be the hallmark of the 1950s, namely "obliviousness."

We can start with the positives. How do they work? Consider the case of the Minnesota-based Search Institute's research on what they call the 40 Developmental Assets, an important element in understanding positive psychology [10].

Based upon their research with many tens of thousands of kids across the country, the Search Institute created a list of positive influences on development. The 40 assets are grouped into eight categories: Support, Empowerment, Boundaries and Expectations, Constructive Use of Time, Commitments to Learning, Positive Values, Social Competencies, and Positive Identity.

If you look at what is included in the "Boundaries and Expectations" you find a very 1950s agenda, for example, "Family has clear rules and consequences, and monitors the young person's whereabouts." And, "School provides clear rules and consequences." And, "Neighbors take responsibility for monitoring young people's behavior." And, "Parent(s) and other adults model responsible behavior." And, "Young person's best friends model responsible behavior." And, "Both parent(s) and teachers encourage the young person to do well."

The emphasis on the old fashioned concept of kids being embedded within a positive structure of adult authority is clear here, but it is also evidenced in other asset clusters. For example, within Constructive Use of Time we find the following asset: "Young person spends three or more hours per week in sports, clubs, or organizations at school and/or in the community organizations." Among Positive Values we find "Young person accepts and takes personal responsibility." Within Positive Identity we find "Young person reports that 'my life has a purpose,'" and among Support is "Young person receives support from three or more nonparent adults."

It is all very 1950s, but it still works! The more of these assets kids have in their lives, the more likely it is that they avoid commonly acknowledged problems like substance abuse and violence. Based upon studies involving about 150,000 6–12th graders, the Search Institute found that with respect to violence, for example, only 6% of kids with 31–40 assets demonstrate a problem with violence, but among kids with 0–10 assets the figure is 61%. The results for substance abuse parallel the findings for violence: 38% for those with 0–10 assets vs. 1% for those with 31–40 use illicit drugs, and for problem alcohol use it is 45 vs. 3%.

On the positive side, for kids with 0–10 assets, the rate of school success is 7%, maintaining good health is 25%, and for delaying gratification 27%, whereas for kids with 31–40 assets, the corresponding numbers are 53, 88, and 72%. All three of these positives represent old fashioned values that are validated by modern research, in the sense that good things flow to people who succeed in school, who cultivate health, and who are able to postpone gratification for later payoffs. All three are linked to the foundations of positive psychology as seen from the perspective of Seligman and others who have researched the origins of enduring happiness and fulfillment in life.

One of the negative correlates of too few assets discovered in the Search Institute's research is the link to sexual activity prior to age 15. This might seem simply like a bias, in the sense that the age of sexual onset is *only* a matter of values, meaning that younger and older onset of sexual activity are not fundamentally different in the meaning and impact on child development, but only reflect the social conventions of a particular time and place. While that may be true (and certainly for parents and most other adults in the 1950s it was a matter of value), it is more than that, at least in North America, because research reveals that becoming sexually active prior to age 15 is correlated with a variety of other measures that clearly have negative consequences for human development. These include lower levels of academic achievement and higher rates of unwanted pregnancies, sexually transmitted diseases, multiple sexual partners, and involvement in other risky behaviors, such as substance use and delinquency [11]. For early onset of sexual activity, the numbers are 34% for 0–10 assets and 3% for 31–40 assets [10].

While much has changed since the 1950s in the lives of kids, what parents say they want for their children is mostly the same now as it was then. Over the last 10 years, I have had occasion to ask parents all around the country, "If you could choose to give your kids good character or $1,000,000, which would you choose?" They are unanimous in choosing "good character," at least in public (which means at least they know the right answer to this question, even if they don't know how to achieve it or actually do things in and with their families that work against achieving that goal). The links between having Developmental Assets and demonstrating the components of character is clear in the Search Institute's research. The more assets kids have in their lives, the more likely that they are living up to the kind of ideals their parents and teachers hope for.

An inspection of the rest of the 40 Developmental Assets (see them at http://www.search-institute.org) reveals a great deal of congruence with life as it was lived in the 1950s (at least in the mainstream of the middle class families to which 90% claimed membership). This is not surprising, given the Search Institute's founder, Peter Benson. I know Peter, and he is, in many ways, a 1950s kind of guy – solid, prosocial, and living a life of purposeful commitments to community, family, and youth development.

Some of the assets are clearly "post 1950s" concerns – most notably, "Young person has knowledge of and comfort with people of different cultural/racial/ethnic backgrounds." And most of these assets are timeless as aspirations, e.g. "Young person can resist negative peer pressure and dangerous situations." But many of them are assets that the social environment supported better in the 1950s than it does now, with the myriad of powerfully corrupting forces, temptations, and demands that distract kids from attending to things like doing their homework, reading, being optimistic about the future, staying home on school nights, and interacting with your family. In this sense, the 1950s were a more positive time in which to grow up, even though some kids in the 1950s did not have these assets or the positive attributes they predict, and many kids today do have the assets and the positive attributes. Long live the 1950s…at least in this respect.

As I said before, I want to see what was good and true about that era, as a way of recognizing in place some of the key elements of positive psychology. At the same time, I want to have a perspective that will allow me see to the secret wrongs, the unspoken pain, and the lack of awareness that were as characteristic of the era as well its simple benefits and pleasures. I want to use this reflection on growing up in the 1950s as an opportunity to consider the pros and cons of what I consider to be the hallmark of the 1950s, namely "obliviousness." Perhaps I can start with some thoughts about growing up in general, with a special focus on the ways in which positive elements nurture children, knowing full well that terrible things do happen to children and their parents, the challenge of which I will return to in the next chapter, when I deal with trauma.

What is the concept that permits a transition from the pros of the 1950s to the cons? I think it is the fundamental issue of acceptance vs. rejection. Human beings evolved to thrive in conditions where they are accepted and languish when rejected. This is one of the few "universals" in child development. Rejection is about actions that send a message "you are not good" and thus offer a negative definition of self to a child. As anthropologist Ronald Rohner documented in his 1975 book *They Love Me, They Love Me Not* [12], and in hundreds of studies since then, rejection is universally a psychological malignancy, an emotional cancer that cuts across societies and cultures to disrupt development and distort behavior. Children and youth thrive on acceptance, and 25% of all the bad behavior and disrupted development observed in children the world over can be attributed to the experience of rejection in place of acceptance [13].

Thus, one way to assess the pros and cons of the 1950s as a positive environment is to focus on the whos and whys of acceptance and rejection: who was accepted, who was rejected, and why. I think it is clear that acceptance in the 1950s was enhanced by many of the fundamental conditions of life. More kids lived in two parent families, and this alone tends to increase acceptance because it spares kids from asking a series of questions that often do get asked – even if secretly – by kids for whom parental absence is an issue. These questions include, "Why didn't my father love me enough to stay?" and "Why didn't my mother love me enough to stay married to my father?" and the more general "What's wrong with me?"

Seligman is aware of this, noting that "children of stable marriages mature more slowly in sexual terms, they have more positive attitudes toward potential mates and are more interested in long-term relationships than are the children of divorce," (p. 188) [9]. Of course, what seems to be at stake here is just what we mean by "stable marriages." Because people were more likely to "stay together for the kids" and to hide their adult problems from their kids ("the children are watching"), even marriages that were deeply troubled (as I eventually understood my parents' to be) were perceived by children as "stable." As the decades passed, however, the transparency of marital problems between parents became ever more evident – through increasingly true-to-life portrayals in the mass media to which children had access, changing mores that encouraged parents to be more open with their children, and the fact that more and more children actually experienced the divorce of their parents.

Beyond families, the general level of social competition in the 1950s was lower than it is now in many ways (at least for groups not experiencing overt discrimination based on their identity). This promoted acceptance. Even though poverty existed, the overall level of economic inequality in the society was so much lower than it is today. This promoted a sense of acceptance because there was less evidence in your face that some people were better than others because they were more successful economically. Consider as an example the fact that today the ratio of CEO to worker salaries is about 250 to 1, whereas when these data were first collected in the mid-1960s it was 25 to 1 (and presumably was at least that low in the 1950s) [14].

What is more, the nature of day-to-day life was much less dependent upon being able to buy "cultural equipment" such as media technology, expensive clothes, and enrichment experiences. As a result, it was easier for kids (and adults, for that matter) to feel accepted because they had what was normal. When no one has a cell phone, a DVD player, an iPod, and cable TV, no one feels left out (and thus rejected) for not having these things. It was easier then to be "normal." I think often of a boy I interviewed in the mid-1990s who asked me, "Dr. G when you were coming up, were you poor or regular." If these are the choices, then being poor means being "irregular." This is much more a contemporary problem than a problem of the 1950s when most of us were in the same boat, even if some of us had better seats.

At least on the surface, and in the direct experience of most children, the 1950s were generally less socially "toxic" than the present [15]. Social toxicity refers to the extent to which the social environment is psychologically poisonous, in the sense that it contains serious threats to the development of identity, competence, moral reasoning, trust, hope, and the other features of personality and ideology that make for success in school, family, work, and the community, all the elements that Seligman identified as core components of positive psychology.

Like physical toxicity, social toxicity can be fatal in the form of suicide, homicide, drug-related and other life style-related preventable deaths. But mostly, it results in diminished "humanity" in the lives of children and youth by virtue of leading them to live in a state of degradation, whether they know it or not. It is the antithesis of what positive psychology aspires to foster in kids and their parents, teachers, and neighbors.

What are the social and cultural poisons that are psychologically equivalent to lead and smoke in the air, PCB's in the water, and pesticides in the food chain? We can see social toxicity in the values, practices, and institutions that breed feelings of fear about the world, feelings of rejection by adults inside and outside the family, exposure to traumatic images and experiences, absence of adult supervision, and inadequate exposure to positive adult role models. These feelings and experiences arise from being embedded in a shallow materialist culture, being surrounded with negative and degrading media messages, and being deprived of relationships with sources of character in the school, the neighborhood, and the larger community.

Were the 1950s less socially toxic? It's hard to know for sure, of course. At the very least I think we can say that there were more intact social systems around families in the form of neighborhoods and schools to cover up and compensate for whatever families lacked themselves. Today, the fragmentation of these social structures allows social toxins to reach children directly, without effective buffering by powerful protective adults. The explosion of communications technologies also plays a role, both allowing the rapid spread of socially toxic cultural forces and sometimes exaggerating their existence and impact. This is because the staid "news" of an older era has been replaced by a no holds barred approach that relies upon fear mongering, salaciousness, celebrity worship, and obliterating the boundaries between "mature adult" topics and the access of children and youth to everything under the sun (and under every rock as well). This is what I see most clearly when I compare growing up in the 1950s with growing up today, and this difference speaks to the pillars of positive psychology and how they are or are not promoted in the social environments in which human development takes place.

The 1950s offered many children a socially benign environment. The structure of benevolent adult authority was relatively intact, at least when compared with the world of twenty-first century America. Adults were adults and kids were kids. The social contract between children and adults was intact and in force: Children will live in their world (under the direct supervision of empowered adults); adults will live in theirs (mostly out of sight from the innocent eyes of children). Adults were in charge and in return took responsibility for protecting children.

There was a high level of public trust; at the beginning of the 1960s, when asked to respond to the question, "Can you count on the government to do the right thing most of the time" some 80% of American adults said, "yes" [16]. Now it is less than 20%. There were only three networks at the time, and television was a trusted force for mainstream reasonableness. This was the time when the late CBS news anchor Walter Cronkite became "the most trusted man in America."

When compared with what had happened before and what has happened since, there was a high level of family stability: 90% of kids lived in two parent families, compared with 68% in 2002 (and only 24% of all households were composed of a married couple with their own children) [17]. As we shall see shortly, all this close-by stability in the lives of kids did not mean that life was free of fear when it came to the world beyond the home, the safe neighborhood, and the safe school (which, of course, for some children weren't safe either, as our belated recognition of child maltreatment, neighborhood violence, and bullying at school have brought to societal consciousness).

The positive side of the 1950s derived from the socially benign character of life for most Americans, as evidenced by the many ways in which the 40 Developmental Assets were nurtured, encouraged, supported, and even demanded by the institutions and ethos of that era. The negative flows from the fact that the various isms and prejudices that embody rejection were still in full flower in the 1950s, and this contributed to an obliviousness that hurt those who were not inside the mainstream circle.

Racism was still an overwhelming force in communicating rejection to racial minorities – most notably African-Americans, who were still legally left out and actively rejected until the Civil Rights Movement broke down some barriers in the following decade (a process that was not even complete with the election of Barrack Obama as President in 2008). Religious sectarianism was still strong in the 1950s; it was not until 1960 that a Catholic could overcome this prejudice and John Kennedy could be elected President. Even in the twenty-first century, it seems implausible that an atheist or agnostic or Buddhist or Hindu or Muslim could manage that feat. But the fanatical rage of the "Religious Right" was not visible on the national scene for the most part in the 1950s. Most of the sociocultural rejections of "traditional American values" were mostly unchallenged in the 1950s, and that is one of the costs of obliviousness in that era that must be reckoned with along with the sources of acceptance for those who were inside the mainstream circle of the time.

Even for those of us who were inside the mainstream circle the issue of obliviousness cut close. For example, hospitalized children in some communities could only be visited once a week by family members. No one seemed to be aware of the negative effect this had on children (and parents). Schools were committed to a "one size fits all" approach (and few people seemed concerned about or even aware of differences in "learning styles"). Communities were set up for the convenience of two parent, one breadwinner families (and few seemed to think about how unwieldy, inconvenient, and unwelcoming this was to single parent or two bread-winner families who could not take care of their business – such as banking and shopping and dentist appointments – between nine and five Monday through Friday). There was less interest and awareness of our inner lives in general, including children, in a way that now seems sometimes almost barbaric. I have a family story that captures this well.

When I was 11 years old, my mother gave birth to my sister Karen. She was a difficult baby, and she developed colic. This meant she started crying every day in the late afternoon and did not stop until sometime in the evening. Since my father – a musician – worked evenings, he was not there during the difficult hours each day. Being the hyperresponsible 1950s boy that I was (making tea for my mother every night was one of my jobs and scrubbing the kitchen floor each Friday was another), I helped with my sister – carrying her around, sometimes for hours at a time.

But my mother bore the brunt of my sister's colic, of course. This came to a head late one afternoon after my dad had left for work, when my mother went up stairs and returned a few minutes later with a packed suitcase. Handing me the baby she said, "take care of your sister," and walked out the front door. There I was, an 11-year-old boy holding a screaming baby, while my mother walked out the door with her suitcase. She returned 15 min later – after she had gotten as far as the corner and had herself a good cry. But these events are not the point of the story.

The point of the story is that this event was always defined within my family – and as I related it to others – as a *positive* story, a testimonial to what a mature and responsible child I was. It was a story almost emblematic of the oblivious 1950s, when people just carried on and did not recognize, let alone dwell, on the dimensions of their inner lives. The story was even told many years later a couple of times when I was being introduced as a professional child psychologist before giving a lecture on child protection, with words to the effect that "and ever since then people have been asking Jim to take care of their children."

I used to interpret that story as a badge of honor, something of which I was proud. It was my wife Claire who helped me see – and thus feel – the horror of this story. How must I have felt to be left holding the baby while my mother walked out the door? For decades, the answer to that question was "I have no idea what I felt then." It was not until Claire offered me another interpretation that I began to have any access to the feelings of that 11-year-old boy in 1958. I must have been terrified, but there was no room for that feeling then – and in the decades that followed until I began to open my heart and reclaim my childhood as the ethos of the post-1950s era began to penetrate my psyche. The 1950s did not prepare kids to be introspective. They cultivated obliviousness instead.

Of course, not everyone is as primed for obliviousness as I was. Some individuals have an extraordinary sensitivity that transcends the blinders that a culture of obliviousness tries to place on their heart's eyes. Others, like me, are particularly prone to obliviousness because our neurological system makes it difficult to develop empathy, to appreciate intuitively the point of view others, read body language, and understand the emotional dimensions of communication.

Back in the 1950s, when I was growing up no one had a name for this pattern and certainly did not recognize its roots in brain function. Back in the 1950s, no one was able to tell me that I existed on the border of Asperger's syndrome. Asperger's in men like me (it is more common in males than females) includes difficulty in friendships, communication problems and an inability to understand social rules and body language. It is understood now to be along the continuum of neurological sensitivity and impairment that ends with autism at its extreme end [18].

Until recently, this condition was not known outside the obscure work of the Austrian psychiatrist and pediatrician Hans Asperger (who first "diagnosed" it in the mid-1940s, and after whom the term is named) [18]. It wasn't until the 1980s that the term was introduced to the English-speaking world, and over the decades since has found a significant place in efforts to understand why some of us develop as we do, "clueless" to some of life's important emotional realities. As I mentioned before, it wasn't until I was 20 that I realized my parents had been separated when I was 3; it wasn't until I was past 60 that I realized I verged on Asperger's. I had long appreciated that I experienced the world differently from most people. Claire had helped me see this – as she had many other things. I had heard and used the term as a psychologist. But I had resisted the realization that there was a personal connection to my life.

It was not until I sat and watched the film "Adam" in 2009 that it all came together for me in a shocking realization that the pattern of internal and social experiences that I had been experiencing all my adult life, when put together brought me close to the conditions of Asperger's. In the life of main character in "Adam" I could see enough of myself to finally make the connection (although it was clear that my condition was far less extreme than Adam's).

Of the characteristics said to be common in Asperger's, I think the following apply to me particularly: Above average intelligence, difficulties in empathizing with others, problems with understanding another person's point of view, hampered conversational ability, and "specialized fields of interest." But I have had a lot going for me that has obscured this problem, and some of the obscuring is related to growing up as I did in the 1950s.

For one thing, I was exposed to a lot of "social skills training" (which clinicians now believe is one way, perhaps the only way, to improve the functioning of people with Asperger's as a substitute for learning the ropes of human relationships the way "normal" people do) [19]. My parents and my teachers taught me how to behave, inculcating "good manners," "polite conversation," "being responsible," and "participating in prosocial activities." There was a kind of 1950s ruthlessness to this, of course: my shyness and tendency to get easily overwhelmed by a lot of social contact was not an acceptable excuse for social withdrawal. When it came to participating in the social life of my community, school, and neighborhood, it was sink or swim. My mother particularly was of the "suffering builds character" school of child rearing – as were most parents in the 1950s.

In part because of the social skills training I was exposed to "inadvertently" as a child, and the fact that my "specialized" expertise was in human behavior and development (not astronomy or mathematics) I learned to "pass" as a child, even becoming a leader among my peers (from starting a club of kids in my neighborhood in elementary school to being elected vice-president of my senior class in high school to serving as president of my undergraduate student government). This social skills training allowed me to succeed in the professional world and in the few friendships I developed and (barely) maintained. Instead of focusing on something like astronomy or numbers (an Asperger's dead giveaway), I have cultivated an intense interest in people – even though I have always had a studied detachment about them. I am a good academic psychologist: my professional success is testament to this.

Once I realized that I have Asperger's traits, I began to see many otherwise puzzling attributes in a new light. For example, I think it is somehow connected to the way I respond more to "fictional" emotional accounts of human lives than "documentary" ones. Reality shows seem emotionally pale to me in comparison with dramas. I now realize this is because the fictional accounts provide more vivid clues to me on what the action means emotionally, whereas often the documentaries assume that the viewer will have an intuitive empathic response. Thus, the fictional accounts coach and prompt me, so I know how to respond in an emotionally appropriate way.

I also understand better why I get so tired being in social situations, and sometimes seem aloof when not officially "on" (for example at cocktail parties and receptions). It is exhausting to have to "act," and it is exhausting to be engaged in trying to figure out the socially appropriate response to people because I don't "get" the spontaneous feedback that normally guides a person in social situations. When I am "on stage" (teaching, lecturing, consulting, and telling stories), I am lively, funny, engaging, and full of sympathetic emotion. When I am with young children or dogs I thrive. But adults? Not so much. Having Asperger's traits explains to me how and why there seems to be a neurological basis for my alternating between being aloof and "on" in adult social situations, and generally comfortable with situations in which I can share my childlike inner life with youngsters and canines.

They say that because of having trouble understanding the emotions of others a person with Asperger's may be seen as egotistical, selfish, and uncaring. This is mostly not true of most of "us." I know it is not true of me. Let me make it clear that my intentions are good: I believe I am "a good person." At heart I am a person of light and spirit. I am kind, generous, compassionate, caring, and giving to the degree that I can "figure out" what the kind, generous, compassionate, caring, and giving thing to do would be. But translating my good intentions to socially appropriate good actions is intrinsically a challenge for me, and I fail at it the more "intimate" the situation – for example, as husband, father, and friend. I mostly get better at it as I get "trained" to know the "right thing" to say and do; I'm actually much better at it now than I was years ago. Growing up in the 1950s ironically fed my intrinsic obliviousness in private, while at the same time, it prepared me to transcend it in my public life. How 1950s is that! But there was a profoundly social dimension to the obliviousness cultivated in the 1950s as well.

Where else did it have an effect? It hid the savage costs of racism from even well meaning White people. It hid the costs of sexism from even well-intended men. One of the worst things it did for kids was to ill-prepare them for the reality of same-sex orientation in adult life. Through the 1960s and early 1970s, even the professional psychological community was part of the problem when it came to meeting the needs of gay and lesbian individuals for acceptance (from parents, teachers, peers, and the larger community) [20]. Although it took decades of advocacy to do so, the professional psychological community has acknowledged that whatever we may call the bias against homosexuals, there is no scientific foundation for it [20].

In the 1950s, homosexuals were virtually invisible in public life, despite the fact that most experts think that about 10% of adults were at their core, naturally gay and lesbian then, as they are now. Then, few of us would even recognize a gay or lesbian person if we were in the same room with them – which, of course, we were, little did we know. One of my best friends in college hid his homosexuality from me and the rest of our otherwise tight group of male friends. It pains me to this day that he did not think he could trust even us, his best friends, with the secret. My pain was made intolerable when I learned that some years after we graduated and lost touch he had committed suicide. His invisibility and our obliviousness cost him dearly.

Today, there is less of this invisibility, less of this obliviousness, and the available evidence indicates that this is very much for the better. Research has shown that there is nothing intrinsically unhealthy about being gay or lesbian. The American Psychological Association and the American Psychiatric Association have (finally) validated this fact and argued against therapeutic interventions based solely on sexual orientation [20].

In addition, it turns out that the sexual orientation of parents is trivial in its importance to successful family function when it comes to producing competent, prosocial, well adjusted, and happy offspring. Research demonstrates that other characteristics of parents are much more important in shaping personality and behavior than their sexual orientation. Gay and lesbian parents have been shown to succeed or fail as parents because of other characteristics, characteristics that are unrelated to sexual orientation (and on average, lesbian parents seem to produce kids who are ever better adjusted and more competent than children of heterosexual parents) [21]. Of course, this assumes that the societies and communities in which they live have given up the stigma against gay or lesbian parents, and do not harshly punish them or their children for this irrelevant fact of their sexual identity.

Even professional validation of the normality of same sex orientation did not end homophobic actions, of course. A study of high school students published in 1998 found that in comparison with heterosexual kids, gay, lesbian, and bisexual youth were five times more likely to miss school because they felt unsafe, four times more likely to be threatened with a weapon at school, twice as likely to have their property damaged at school, and three times more likely to require medical treatment after a fight at school (despite the fact that they were four times less likely to be involved in fighting at school) [22]. And, it is still true that openly homosexual individuals are barred from serving in the US military – and they continue to be discharged once their "secret" is officially acknowledged (this even as some military leaders have joined progressive political leaders in arguing for an end to this policy). Bias against homosexuals continues even amidst great cultural progress.

This is evident in the "Secret Lives of Teenagers" study my colleagues and I conducted with students from Cornell University when I taught there for 10 years starting in the mid-1990s [23]. The students were asked about many aspects of their lives – what they thought, what they felt, what they did, and what happened to them – and then asked if their parents were aware of these facts about their lives. With respect to sexual orientation, the results revealed that few parents were aware of their offspring's homosexual orientation. Ten percent of the males revealed that they realized they were gay during high school but 60% said their parents never knew. Among females, 10% revealed that they realized they were lesbians during high school but 90% said their parents never knew. This, I think, is evidence that adolescents with same sex orientations may have feared rejection from their parents in the majority of families, and certainly did not have relationships that would allow open communication on a deep personal level. Of course, overall things are much better today for homosexual humans than they were in the 1950s, when the costs of obliviousness exacted a terrible price from so many perfectly normal souls.

If the traumatic impact of 1950s' obliviousness is exemplified by the experience of gays and lesbians, its benevolent impact is evident in the fact that with each new year after the 1950s ended, children's visual access to scary stuff increased, whether it be horrific violence of war and crime, parental incapacitation, family break up, the clay feet of political leaders, or the sweaty details of sexuality. One of the big challenges families faced in the 1950s was to convey basic emotional messages to children regarding both sexuality in general and their sexual orientation in particular. At its worst, this teaching often conveyed the message, "sex is dirty and disgusting… save it for someone you love." At its best it taught "sex is so important and so powerful that it is best saved for someone you love and are committed to."

To this end, consider this: when eminent sex researchers Masters and Johnson (who studied the "plumbing" of human sexuality as no one had before) were asked about the best form of sex education, they did not recommend graphic sex videos. Instead, they replied with words to the effect that "it is your parents doing the dishes together in the kitchen and mom leans up against dad and he puts his arm around her and she gives him a kiss on the cheek" [24]. There was a lot of that going on in the 1950s – on television and in real-life kitchens.

The message was clear: if you learn about sex in the context of loving commitment, the matters of "plumbing" are easy to learn. But, if all you have is technique divorced from an understanding of the role of loving commitment as a context for sex you will need remedial education to achieve a mature adult experience (and this will likely be manifest in a negative autobiography and stunted spiritual development). I think time has borne out the wisdom of this message.

Whatever the many sexual "hang ups" that parents and other adults taught kids in the 1950s – and there were far too many – this was a time when kids were more likely to learn about the core issues of sex in the way that Masters and Johnson recommended than they are today, when for so many kids the pressing concerns are the fact that your mother and/or father is sleeping with someone who is not your parent, and you are bombarded with explicit sexual messages couched in aggression or shallow materialism to sell products on television, in the movies, in music, and on the internet.

A study led by David Brickman found that young children (age 6–8) who watch prime-time television are substantially more likely to start having sex when they are 12–14 years old than if they don't: "The study found that for every hour the youngest group of children watched adult-targeted content (which also included movies, reality shows, and sports – anything that aired during prime-time viewing hours, 8–11 p.m.) over two sample days, their chances of having sex during early adolescence increased by 33%" [25]. Many prime-time shows are highly sexualized (like one of my favorites CBS's – "Two and Half Men" – that I would never have wanted my children to watch). Even if they aren't, they tend to portray the clay feet of adults, which contributes to breaking down the adult authority that can and does serve as a disincentive to early sexual behavior (as was seen earlier when we looked at the 40 Developmental Assets).

On another note, research suggests that experiences within the family that affect a child's understanding and expectations regarding physical pleasure and pain can affect their sexual development. For example, research reveals a small (but statistically significant) association between physical punishment of children by parents (particularly "loving" parents) and an inclination for sadomasochistic sexual practices in adulthood [26]. And, sexual experiences between adults and children within families can affect subsequent sexual orientation and practices. One of these was open in the 1950s – namely corporal punishment by loving parents. The other was a secret, a very dark secret: researchers working on the issue of child sexual abuse in the 1950s claimed that the prevalence as somewhere between one in a million and one in seven million [27]. Today, the common estimates cluster around one in ten, not because there is more sexual abuse now, but because it was shamefully hidden then. Here is an area where obliviousness was very costly indeed, as is evident in the searing testimony of many adults who were silenced as child victims and have paid the price for that silence ever since.

Another social toxin from the 1950s was the emergence of a low-grade fear of annihilation that was rarely acknowledged in public, but which was an undertone to the generally positive spirit of the times. An ancient text from the Zoroastrian tradition in Persia states, "To live in fear and falsehood is worse than death," and the threat of atomic war provided the impetus to a subterranean culture of fear.

In 1936, when my mother was 12 years old, she and her friends sat in front of her row house in a working class neighborhood of London and the conversation turned to death. "I wonder if I will be alive in 1940?" she wondered, frightened that a serial killer known as "the man with the staring eyes" would make her his next victim and that the Italian invasion of Abbysinia (Ethiopia as it is called today) would escalate to another world war. Her father having fought in World War I less than 20 years earlier, that conflict was a vivid memory in her family. Talking about it 70 years later, my mother now realizes that news of the impending war in Europe was feeding her anxiety about death and that it provided the emotional power of the closer-to-home fear of the killer on the loose.

By 1940, my mother was spending nights in the bomb shelter in the back yard of her family's house and finding her way through the rubble of London under siege from the German air force. In 1943, she forged her parents' names on her application to join the Royal Air Force and became part of the British national security state mobilized to fight the Nazis and protect her homeland.

This carried on into my own life. In 1954, when I was 7 years old, and living in New York City, my teachers drilled us to expect atomic attack at any moment. The import of their words remains with me half a century later: "If you see a bright flash in the sky you must duck under your desk immediately before the blast can blow out the windows of the classroom" ("and decapitate you" was left unsaid, but was clearly implicit in the threat). As a result, I carried around the conviction that the next flash of light in the sky I saw would mean the long awaited atomic attack from the Soviet Union on the American homeland.

After all, the most trusted adults in our lives warned us about this "fact" through these often repeated "duck and cover" drills, and underscored the grim reality of it all by giving us dog tags with our blood type and names on them – "in case." The 1952 film "Atomic City" contains a scene in which a young boy sitting at the kitchen table says to his mother who is doing the dishes, "Mom, if I grow up..." His uncertainty about the future was on our minds as children too. One way we responded was by indulging in military fantasies. After school and on weekends, my friends and I played "army," in our play reflecting the increasing militarization of American life that came with the Cold War.

Then in 1962, when I was 15, the Cuban Missile Crisis brought me once again to a sense of impending doom. American and Soviet forces were on a state of high alert, and subsequent revelations of documents and first-hand accounts by government officials on both sides reveal that the world was literally on the verge of an exchange of nuclear weapons. It was well-grounded fear, not panicky paranoia that drove my parents and our neighbors to stock up on groceries and discuss the relative merits of various types of bomb shelters – particularly those that could be built in the back yard versus those that could be fashioned out of a corner of the basement. In the years that followed I was eager to attend West Point so that I might join the Army to serve my country and protect the homeland in the great struggle against the Evil Empire. I failed the physical for West Point, and so joined Army ROTC in college, continuing on a military track until I had a pacifist awakening one night when I played the role of "the enemy" in a mock battle and I realized what all the words of glory hid, that it was about killing and being killed (but that's another story).

Four decades after the Cuban Missile Crisis, and in the wake of 9/11, my own young adult children worried about going to New York City or Washington, DC on holidays for fear of a terrorist attack, and I worry about returning to the Middle East again where I have been often since the mid-1980s for fear of unwittingly becoming a victim in the struggle there. Once again, homeland insecurity seems of paramount importance as a public issue: a survey done in July 2005 found that Americas rated the threat of terrorism as the nation's number one problem [28].

Despite the challenges parents of the 1950s faced with the rise of atomic war as a threat, I believe that they had an easier time of it when it came to protecting children, than I did as a parent in the 1980s and 1990s, than do parents in the world of the twenty-first century. For one thing, the flow of information to children 50 years ago was under relatively tight and mostly benign control. To be sure, this control had a down side (e.g., in its narrow portrayal of females and ethnic and racial minorities and the absence of people with other than heterosexual orientation). But on the plus side, television was effectively censored when it came to the sweaty details of gross adult sex and vivid violence.

There was a strong sense that "children are watching," which meant that adults should forego the pleasure and titillation of explicit sexuality on the screen. Of course, this censorship limited the ability of television and the movies to deal with some adult subjects, but in retrospect I don't think the cost was too great. Themes of sexuality, infidelity, debilitating illness, depression, suicide, and murder could be presented, but in a manner that seems muted, dignified, and subtle by today's "let it all hang out" standards.

There was violence, but it was highly stylized and sanitized. The "bad guys" were only moderately nasty, and the "good guys" subscribed to a strict code of honorable conduct. In the television environment of the 1950s, even the child of a negligent parent was at little risk sitting in front of the television set, because the narrow range of available images and themes was tightly controlled by the adults who made and broadcast the programming. The same was true for movies. There was a systematic cover up of the dark side of American history, of course: no images of how the Native-American population was slaughtered, how African-Americans were lynched, how women were victims of domestic violence, how children were abused and neglected, how animals were treated with callous cruelty. But in addition, there was a kind of security here.

But this sense of security, it turned out, was in some ways false. For example, research on the impact of televised violence indicates that its effect on increasing aggressive behavior by child viewers is equivalent to the effect of smoking on lung cancer – namely that it accounts for about 10–15% of the variation [29]. In this sense, violent television is a social toxin. The rise of toxic television began almost coincidentally with the start of broadcasting itself, although there can be little doubt that the TV of the 1950s was benign by today's standards, at least in the potentially traumatic and toxic nature of the images it presented.

The media technology of the 1950s also worked to the advantage of children. Special effects were primitive and not likely to produce the kind of visual trauma associated with contemporary images. The cumbersome quality of visual recording technology – limited for the most part to film – reduced to negligible the possibility that real-life horrific events would be made available visually to the television and movie viewer, including the child viewer.

Today, the ubiquitous availability of video recording means that much of what is horrible to see will be made available for the seeing, and usually by children as readily as by adults. Consider the horror of the attack on Pearl Harbor in 1941 versus the attack on the World Trade Center 60 years later. The former was visually witnessed by a relative handful of children; the latter was seen via videotape by virtually every child in America – over and over again, in many cases. Repeat this for every violent and traumatic image over and over again, from the big events such as plane crashes to the little events such as ritual beatings purveyed over local television news as well as over You-Tube and other internet sites that cater to kids.

This exposure to traumatic imagery is one important feature of the social toxicity which compounds the problem of parents and other caring adults in helping children deal with growing up in the age of terror. But it is not the only element.

Studies from around the world and in North America as well document that parents who are able to see and hear the feelings of their children, and respond respectfully and warmly to these feelings are most likely to produce emotionally healthy children [23]. Is this any more true in the age of terror than at any other time? I think the answer is a qualified "yes." Let me explain. The challenge of raising successful children does contain universal elements, but all parenting takes place in a particular social and cultural context, and the exigencies of each human ecology shape the tasks parents face and how they successfully translate their love into effective child rearing.

One of the more interesting findings to come out of research directed at children in the wake of 9/11 was a small study conducted by the people who produce the Sesame Street program for television – The Children's Television Workshop [30]. The investigators asked about 100 children, ages 6–11 years to fill out a booklet called "All About Me." The children wrote essays and included pictures. The older children, 9–11 years old also used disposable cameras to take pictures of important settings in their lives such as "the wise one" and "the safe place." Ironically, the children reported more fears and anxiety about violence in June 2000 than they did in the weeks immediately following the 9/11 attacks. How could that be? The authors speculate that in the immediate aftermath of 9/11 parents were in a heightened state of awareness about the need to attend to their children's emotional lives, and as a result were more likely to ask about and listen to their children's inner lives. As one of the researchers (Susan Royer) put it: "Most importantly, when things are 'normal,' children seem to feel most alone and helpless in their fear, and unlike Code Orange times, parents can be clueless about kids' anxiety, and kids know that" [30].

This study is quite consistent with psychological research over several decades as well as the insights of psychotherapists and parent educators: empathic parenting is both crucial to the well being of children and in short supply on a day-to-day basis [4]. Director Steven Spielberg acknowledged in an interview that he approached making the 2005 film "War of the Worlds" differently because of 9/11 than he would have before [31]. But there was more to the interview than this point. Spielberg recalls the 1951 science fiction film "Invaders from Mars" as the most disturbing of the many such films he viewed as a child. Why? Because in the film aliens tamper with a young boy's parents – implanting devices in their necks that allow the aliens to control and manipulate them and in so doing turn them away from their child. As Spielberg sees it, this is the primal fear of childhood, that your parents are not your parents, that they will turn away from you because they are under the control of alien forces. This is why "Invasion from Mars" worked. It is why Spielberg saw it five times. I saw it twice, and it left indelible memories for both of us. The 1950s were a time of relatively stable family life – whatever their faults, your parents were likely to continue to function as your parents. In today's world, this reassurance is missing for most kids (even those who do live with their parents) and the primal fear that Spielberg spoke of is an all too real one for children and youth.

Having said that, though, and although it pales in comparison with today's issues, the 1950s could have been a scary time for sensitive children, what with the repeated warnings of the impending atomic doom that we received from our parents, our teachers, the burgeoning science fiction movie genre, and some of our political leaders. What we needed then (but mostly did not receive) and what children need now (and may well be more likely to get in our much more psychologically sophisticated era) was and is intelligent empathy on the part of parent, and teachers, and every other adult in the lives of children, for that matter. This bodes well for a positive psychology of childhood.

Whatever the modern age is, it is not oblivious in the sense that we were in the 1950s. Perhaps one reason that mainstream psychologists in the 1950s did not study happiness and other positive themes in their research was that they took these things for granted. They bought into the foundation for optimism: overestimating the positive and underestimating the negative, seeing the objectively half full glass as subjectively full. But this optimism came at a price, the price of obliviousness. Awareness may be painful in many ways, but it is the only path to enlightenment. Challenge can be growth inducing, even the ultimate challenge to awareness, namely trauma. If it is met with a positive psychology, even trauma can contribute to the flowering of the best of the human condition, as we shall see in the next chapter.

References

1. http://geography.about.com/od/populationgeography/a/babyboom.htm.
2. http://ezinearticles.com/?Impact-of-Baby-Boomers-on-American-Society&id=932508.
3. http://www.pbs.org/now/politics/middleclassoverview.html.
4. Garbarino, J. (2008) Children and the dark side of human experience: Confronting global realities and rethinking child development. New York: Springer.
5. Bronfenbrenner, U. (1970) Two worlds of childhood. New York: Sage.
6. Bronfenbrenner, U. (1979) The ecology of human development. Cambridge, MA: Harvard University Press.
7. Sammeroff, A. Seifer, R. Barocas, R. Zax, M. and Greenspan, S. (1987) Intelligence quotient scores of 4 year old children: Socio environmental risk factors. Pediatrics, 79, 343–350.
8. Peter De Vries (n.d.). BrainyQuote.com. Retrieved June 29, 2010, from BrainyQuote.com Web site: http://www.brainyquote.com/quotes/quotes/p/peterdevri136826.html.
9. Seligman, M. (2004) Authentic happiness. New York: Free Press.
10. http://www.search-institute.org.
11. Sheier, L. A. and Crosby, R. (2003) Correlates of sexual experience among a nationally representative sample of alternative high school students. The Journal of School Health, 73, 197–200.
12. Rohner, R. (1975) They love me, they love me not. New Haven, CT: Human Area Files Press.
13. Rohner, R. Khalequew, A. and Cournoyer, D. E. (2005) Parental acceptance-rejection: Theory, methods, cross-cultural evidence, and implications. Ethos, 33 (3), 299–334.
14. http://www.epi.org/economic_snapshots/entry/webfeatures_snapshots_20060621/.
15. Garbarino, J. (1995) Raising children in a socially toxic environment. San Francisco: Jossey-Bass.
16. Putnam, R. (2001) Bowling alone: The collapse and revival of American community. New York: Putnam.
17. http://www.childtrendsdatabank.org/.
18. Attwod, T. (2008) The complete guide to Asperger's syndrome. London: Jessica Kingsley.

19. Baker, J. (2003) Social skills training for children and adolescents with Asperger's syndrome and social-communication problems. Shawnee Mission, KS: Autism Asperger Publishing Company.
20. http://www.apa.org/helpcenter/sexual-orientation.aspx.
21. http://www.webmd.com/mental-health/news/20051012/study-same-sex-parents-raise-well-adjusted-kids.
22. Garbarino, J. and deLara, E. (2002) And words can hurt forever: Protecting adolescents from bullying, harassment, and emotional violence. New York: Free Press.
23. Garbarino, J. and Bedard, C. (2001) Parents under siege. New York: Free Press.
24. Masters, W. Johnson, V. and Kolodny, R. (1997) Human sexuality. New York: Allyn and Bacon.
25. http://www.childrenshospital.org/newsroom/Site1339/mainpageS1339P1sublevel528.html.
26. Straus, M. and Donnelly, D. (1994) Beating the devil out of them. New York: Lexington Books.
27. Finkelhor, D. (1986) Sourcebook on child sexual abuse. New York: Sage.
28. http://www.aei.org/article/24492.
29. Bushman, B. J. and Anderson, C. A. (2001). Media violence and the American public: Scientific facts versus media misinformation. The American Psychologist, 56, 477–489.
30. http://www.apa.org/monitor/may03/everyday.aspx.
31. http://www.rd.com/the-truth-behind-spielbergs-war-of-the-worlds/article14939.html.

Chapter 3
Nine Bad Things That Almost Happened, and Many More That Did: Getting to the Other Side of Trauma

Some years ago I listened to "Prairie Home Companion" radio host Garrison Keillor tell a folksy tale about how mostly the bad things that could happen don't. As I recall, the story revolved around him being up a ladder fixing a gutter or something else on the roof when he slipped and fell. He commented on the fact that he might have fallen on something hard or sharp and injured himself severely, but he didn't, and used the occasion to reflect on how so many of the bad things in life that could happen generally don't.

The story made quite an impression on me – in part because I myself had recently fallen from a ladder on my own roof and landed unhurt. But thinking back on it, I was drawn to the idea of how different life is for people when and if the bad things that could happen really do happen. It's one of those "there are two kinds of people…" kind of thing. One kind is most of us, most of the time, while the other is those to whom really bad things really do happen. Much of my professional life has been taken up with understanding this second group, but my personal life has been much more a matter of being part of the first group.

Bad Thing #1: In 1949, when I was 2 years old, my father was working as a musician in Chicago – at the Drake Hotel. My young mother and I stayed back in New York, in a small apartment on West 95th Street. As the story is told, one morning I awakened before my mother, who was then and is today a heavy sleeper – (one day, many years later, my father insisted that we see how long she would sleep if no one woke her up in the morning, but by 4 o'clock that afternoon we could not stand it any longer and woke her up). That morning in 1949, while she slept, I made my way out the living room window so that I could stand on the ledge of the tiny balcony and talk to the cats in the courtyard five stories below.

Soon, our neighbors detected me perched precariously, risking death on the pavement below, and pounded on our apartment door; my mother finally awakened and ordered me back into the apartment. "No," I replied and continued my conversation with the cats below, oblivious to the danger. "Your Daddy sent you a present from Chicago," she countered. "OK," I said, beaming, and made my way back through the window. She proceeded to nail the window shut, and life went on. *That year in the United States about 150 children died, and some 4,000 were treated in emergency rooms because of falling out of windows* [1].

J. Garbarino, *The Positive Psychology of Personal Transformation:*
Leveraging Resilience for Life Change, DOI 10.1007/978-1-4419-7744-1_3,
© Springer Science+Business Media, LLC 2011

Bad Thing #2: A year after I didn't fall off the terrace from the fifth floor of our building, my mother took me on an extended trip to England to visit her family. My parents had met during World War II in London, where my Italian-American father-to-be was serving in the US Army as a soldier-musician and my English mother-to-be was in the Women's Royal Air Force as a teletypist. As the story goes, they met at a dance (although at the moment of first contact she was sitting by herself at a table, she was actually with another man). Dashing young American soldier with soulful eyes that he was, Ray Garbarino was on the prowl – as I suspect was my flirtatious mother-to-be. His opening line was "What's a pretty girl like you doing here all by herself?" Her reply was, "Actually, I'm here with someone." Despite this false start, my mother-to-be fell in love with my father-to-be's soulful saxophone playing, and by the time the war ended they were married. In the meantime, while they courted, she was reassigned as a teletype operator to a base outside London, and he went ashore in France a week and a half after D-Day in June 1944, as a member of his Regimental band and carried his rifle and saxophone across Europe and into Germany (with being caught up in the Battle of the Bulge the most horrifying part of the experience).

So in 1950, when my mother and I boarded the ocean liner Mauritania in New York City to sail to England, it could have been construed as a simple visit by a homesick young English woman and her American son. Indeed, that is what I thought it was for nearly 20 years afterward. We stayed 6 months in England and then (I am told) returned to New York because I "missed my father." What I realized nearly 20 years later was that my parents had nearly undertaken a permanent separation to be followed by a divorce. Whatever her reasons for doing so – her shame about divorce? her missing my father? her fear of making it on her own? *me* missing my father? – I was spared the difficult experience of being a child growing up in a single parent household, being a "child of divorce," and experiencing "father absence." Not long after we returned to New York, my mother discovered she was pregnant with what would turn out to be my brother John, and the issue of separation was put on hold indefinitely. *Nearly 400,000 children experienced divorce the year that my parents almost separated permanently in 1950. For most of them it was a shock, a terrible emotional wrench, a major social dislocation, and a source of shame and fear, an enduring "risk factor" to their development that often reverberated through the rest of their lives* [2].

Bad Thing #3: It was the summer of 1958, and my 7-year-old younger brother John was invited to join his friend Jonathan Tannenbaum, another boy, and Jonathan's mother on an outing to the beach – Jones Beach, a popular ocean destination not far from our home on Long Island, outside New York City. The Tannenbaums were friends of our family, and it was not unusual for John to spend time with them. A trip to the ocean was always a treat, so he was eager to go. But our mother had something else planned, and John could not go. Later that day we heard the news that Jonathan and the other boy had drowned in the surf when a big wave knocked them off their feet and they were swept out to sea. I recall going to Jonathan's wake with my father, John being too young to attend. Sometime later, Jonathan's parents divorced – as do many couples who lose a child, particularly when issues of blame and guilt tear them apart. *That year about 1,400 American children died or suffered severe permanent neurological damage from drowning, but our John was not one of them, and life went on* [3].

Bad Thing #4: On May 24, 1979 I flew on American Airlines flight #191 out of Chicago. There was nothing unusual about that. For the past 35 years I have done a lot of traveling, and often connected through O'Hare Airport. *But the next day, on May 25, that same flight crashed while taking off from Chicago, killing all 270 passengers and crew (and two people on the ground) [4]. My travel agent checked and informed me that it was not only the same flight but the very same plane I had flown on the day before. Precipitous death of this sort haunts family members for decades, sometimes forever.* Even a brush with the possibility of a plane crashing can unnerve people. One day a couple of years later, a commuter flight into Harrisburg, Pennsylvania, declared an emergency because an indicator light showed that its landing gear was not fully deployed. Fire trucks met the flight, but it landed safely. I was on the next flight to depart from Harrisburg (to State College, Pennsylvania) when some of the passengers from the first flight boarded ours to finish their trip. All were badly shaken; some could not stay on the plane, and got off so they could be bused to State College. A couple said that they would never fly again.

Bad Thing #5: My next close encounter with horror came in July 1980. My family and I were spending the summer on a small island in the Adirondacks of northern New York State, as we did every summer for many years. My son Josh was 4 years old, and happy as a clam that he could putter around on the dock and in the shallow water. His familiarity with the place and the relative safety of the shallow water lulled us into a false sense of security. That afternoon we were visited by Josh's Aunt Suzie, along her husband and his 8-year-old daughter. The two children were playing on the dock, and the adults were sipping lemonade on the back porch. Suddenly, the 8-year old ran onto the porch shouting, "Josh is in trouble." I leaped from my chair and ran off the porch in the direction of the lake. As I ran down the dock, I could see only empty lake, no sign of my son. I was preparing to leap into the water as thoughts of finding his body flooded my imagination. Then, as I scanned the water about to jump in from the end of the dock, wondering where to look first, I saw him holding onto the ladder at the end of the dock. He was scared – perhaps as much by my panic as anything else – but alive, not lying dead on the bottom, his lungs full of water. *In 1980, drowning was the number one cause of unintentional death in young children in 18 of the 50 states; hundreds of kids died that year [3].*

Bad Thing #6: One winter night in 1981, while driving on an icy road from the Pittsburgh Airport to my home in State College, Pennsylvania, I came over the crest of a hill to find the scene of a major accident at the bottom of that same hill, nearly blocking the road. As I gently applied the brakes, the car began to skid. The road was icy, and I had no ability to steer. Trusting to fate I tried to guide the car toward the one opening between the damaged vehicles at the bottom of the hill that I could see was potentially wide enough for the car, and I plunged toward the crash scene. Expecting to join the mess of wrecks, I was amazed as my car found its way through the narrow gap unscathed and I continued on my way home. *That same year more than 50,000 people were killed in automobile crashes in the USA [5].* I have been in a few auto accidents – but never injured seriously. Even a minor accident is unnerving; a major crash can leave a person emotionally scarred and even unable to return to driving for a long time.

Bad Thing #7: April 23, 1983. My daughter Joanna almost died this day, but was born instead. I have been through some scary times in my life, but the minutes between when my daughter Joanna was born dead – still and blue as she emerged from her mother's body into the harsh bright light of the delivery room in a small hospital in State College, Pennsylvania – and became *alive* – turning pink and squirmy before my eyes as I searched for the words to tell her mother that the baby was dead – were perhaps the scariest of all.

It was two weeks after the official delivery date and the decision was made to induce labor, as maternal blood pressure was up and the baby was showing signs of distress. Being a second birth, and being induced, contractions came fast and hard, as I sat next to the bed watching the two monitor screens. One told of the impending contractions – and like a good Lamaze coach, it was my job to sound the alert as they began to rise on the screen. The other told of the baby's distress as things wore on – heart rate declining dangerously as the contractions continued. I suppose the baby being late made it a bit crowded in there. Maybe that's just a fantasy. But whatever the cause, the fetal distress was real, real enough to raise the prospect of a C-Section delivery. But before that distressing prospect could be realized, the baby started to come.

Almost unbelievably, the obstetrician (I trust that I am within my rights to call him "the jerk") was annoyed because it was almost 5 o'clock in the afternoon, and his shift was supposed to end at 5. Reluctantly he agreed to recognize the reality that the birth would indeed involve a bit of overtime, and we moved into the delivery room – trailing monitors and nurses. When Joanna emerged she was blue and seemed dead, so I began rehearsing some way to tell her mother. I had wanted a daughter – or a son – to go along with our first born, Josh. I remember feeling profoundly sad and terribly scared. It is amazing how much you can feel and think in a few seconds when in the presence of death. And then they offered the dead blue body some oxygen, and she was alive. It had been a long-standing family joke to say that someone or something rises "Phoenix-like" – as when one emerges from a deep "sleep of the dead," or having fallen playing a game and lain still on the ground a football player raises himself to his feet. But this was no family joke – at least not then, although in future years when the baby was safely grown into childhood it would become one (sort of). The dead baby became alive, and indeed she began to move and even cry a bit – Phoenix-like. She lived, and 27 years later I walked her down the aisle at her wedding. *But across the USA in 1983 year 39,000 babies – more than 100 each day – did die – that is, were still born (meaning they died after reaching at least 20 weeks of gestation)* [6]. *Each was a terrible event that left their parents grieving and often emotionally weakened.* I hate to think what would have become of our family had Joanna not revived that day nearly 30 years ago.

Bad Thing #8: In 1989, my research assistants and I traveled to Nicaragua as part of a project on the impact of war on children. This visit came at a time when the Sandanista government led by Daniel Ortega was in the final stages of its battle with the US-backed Contras. We spent much of our time doing interviews and making site visits in and around the capital city of Managua. One day, however, we made a trip out into the countryside to visit a small town, which had been torn apart by the political violence. Before we left we were warned to be back in Managua before dark because the roads were dangerous at night due to Contra attacks. Getting back before dark seemed logistically simple given the scheduled start time and the length of the drive round trip. Things started to go awry when our driver and guide – a young Sandinista woman – arrived an hour late to pick us up in her government-provided pickup truck.

The day went well – emotionally moving and full of information. As the afternoon wore on and the scheduled time for our return to Managua drew close, however, our guide started to drink with a group of her friends from the local community. Despite our hints, and then pleading, she continued to party, and we grew ever more anxious. By the time we did leave town and get back on the road, the sun was setting, so we made the drive through the danger zone in the darkness we had been warned against. When all was said and done, we did make it back to Managua safely that night. *That year 1,000 civilians were killed in Nicaragua, leaving their families and friends devastated emotionally* [7]. The night after our nerve-wracking trip, a government vehicle traveling the same road we had driven was ambushed, and the occupants were killed.

Bad Thing #9: In 1991 I traveled to Kuwait on behalf of UNICEF, to assess the impact of the Iraqi invasion and occupation on children. A couple of nights after arriving with the UNICEF team, I was on my own with two journalists driving through the dark city – this being just a few days after the Iraqi Army had fled the city. We approached a road block manned by an adolescent boy armed with a rifle – a member of the Kuwaiti Resistance – and he raised his weapon as if to shoot first and ask questions later. The journalists in the front seat began to scream out the Arabic word for "journalist" (Sawiah).

I hid behind the front seat, and for a minute the outcome of the encounter seemed unclear. But then he lowered his weapon and we were able to proceed (to the only hotel in the city with electricity and thus a functioning kitchen where we could get our first hot meal in several days – spaghetti as I recall). *Last year some 70 journalists were killed around the world in acts of political violence or war-related incidents* [8]. *War correspondents are a hearty and brave lot, but once they are actually injured, few are able to continue. The "before" and the "after" are two very different realities.*

Reflecting on all these bad things that have *almost* happened to me and my loved ones over the years, and all the many people to whom they actually did, I am drawn to look anew at what has been a major theme in my professional work for the past three decades: trauma. I do so here to see how it relates to the concepts and ideas of positive psychology, how making sense of the bad things can lead to some good things – if you are fortunate in who your friends are, what resources you have, how your temperament equips you to deal with stress and threat, and how you come out on the other side with a new appreciation for the meaning of life.

The word "trauma" has entered into common usage around the world. That's generally good news, since understanding trauma opens our eyes to how terrible events can transform a life. Of course, like any change of this sort, there is the risk that widespread use of the term "traumatic" may cheapen its core meaning; this is traumatic, that is traumatic. When you hear someone say "I went on a traumatic date" or "That exam was traumatic," and all they really mean is that they were uncomfortable or embarrassed or inconvenienced, the core meaning and significance of "trauma" is diluted.

The real substance of "trauma" is greater and deeper than casual references would allow: trauma is the experience of profound psychological threat. Perhaps the most powerful simple characterization is "an event from which you never fully recover" [9]. Listening to some World War II veterans talk about their experiences with combat on the fiftieth anniversary of D-Day brought that home with a vengeance. More than 50 years later many of the men who experienced that June 6, 1944 are still unable to overcome the horror they felt at the death and suffering – and in some cases the guilt they still feel that they survived while their friends and buddies didn't. Tom Hanks, Steven Spielberg, and their colleagues explored this in their excellent 10-part television series, "Band of Brothers," which chronicles a single US Army unit (E Company – "Easy Company" – of the 2nd Battalion, 506th Parachute Infantry Regiment assigned to the 101st Airborne Division) from basic training through D-Day until the end of the war in Europe, and is based upon historian Stephen Ambrose's book of the same name [10]. Each episode of the television series ends with the real veterans themselves reflecting on their experiences, and the residue of trauma is apparent and abundant in the voices, faces, and tears of many of them.

An Army general commissioned a study of one unit that landed on D-Day and was in combat virtually continuously for the next 2 months. As my friend military psychologist David Grossman tells it in his book "On Killing," when all was said and done, 98% of these soldiers were "psychiatric casualties" by the time 60 days had passed [11]. Most recovered relatively quickly, with short-term rest and therapy – and even returned to their unit. Some never recovered – and could be found in Veteran's Hospitals decades later.

When the General who commissioned the study asked about the 2% who didn't break down – thinking they would be the most psychologically robust individuals – he was told that they all were psychopaths. Why didn't the psychopaths break down after chronic combat that "normal" men found intolerable? The answer lies in the fact that psychopaths are not aroused the way normal people are by witnessing death and injury, and they don't feel the same moral pain that normal people feel about killing. In a sense, the only men who didn't go crazy after 60 days of combat already were!

Judith Herman, a clinical researcher who specializes in sexual abuse cases, uses these words in defining trauma, that to be traumatized is "to come face to face with human vulnerability in the natural world and with the capacity for evil in human nature" [12]. That's powerful and captures the truth of trauma. It is when you experience something bad that breaks down your positive assumptions and conclusions about the world and your place in that world. I know enough to know that had any of the bad things I described earlier actually happened to me, the world would look very different to me – or at least would if I had not successfully digested, processed, and made new sense of the world after the fact. Judith Herman is right on the mark.

Trauma arises when we cannot do two things at once: handle the surge of feelings that floods us when we are faced with horror *and* give meaning to these frightening experiences. To use more conventionally psychological terms, trauma is the *simultaneous* experience of extremely powerful negative feelings ("overwhelming arousal") coupled with thoughts that are beyond normal ideas of human reality ("overwhelming cognitions") [9].

This is one reason why naïve efforts to recover may fail: it requires quieting the arousal, so the ideas can be processed, which is often difficult to accomplish because both the sensations and the ideas can trigger a return of the other, and thus sustain the trauma. Interventions that "immobilize" the arousal (perhaps through drugs or some repetitive behavior like moving your eyes) can allow the psychological space to reprocess the cognitions, and thus lead to improved functioning and even healing [13].

The focus on simultaneously overwhelming arousal and cognitions is contained in the American Psychiatric Association's definition of the psychological consequence of trauma, what they diagnostically label "posttraumatic stress disorder" (PTSD) [14]. PTSD results from encounters with threatening experiences outside the realm of normal experience. This sense of being shaken out of normality is echoed repeatedly in first-person accounts of trauma, like the people to whom really bad things happen (unlike the stories I have told earlier, in which bad things *almost* happen).

Trauma matters in many important ways that shape the individual reality of the people who are traumatized and the social world in which they participate. Before the good things of positive psychology can be reclaimed, the bad things associated with trauma must be dealt with, in part because a traumatic experience that is cognitively overwhelming may stimulate conditions in which the process required to "understand" these experiences itself can have unfortunate and socially disabling side effects. That is, in coping with a traumatic event, a person may be drawn into patterns of behavior, thought, and emotion that are themselves "abnormal" when contrasted with patterns prior to the event, as well as when compared with patterns characterized by untraumatized individuals. In place of optimism there is pessimism; in place of hope there is despair.

But as psychologist Daniel Gilbert has shown in his book *Stumbling on Happiness*, "although more than half the people in the United States will experience a trauma, such as rape, physical assault, or natural disaster in their lifetimes, only a small fraction will ever develop any post-traumatic pathology or require any professional assistance" (pp. 166–167) [15]. Why? Gilbert attributes this resilience to the fact that human brains are inclined to exploit the ambiguity of life's events – finding the positive dimensions of what are ordinarily considered negative events (and, I might note in Gilbert's analysis, vice versa). As we shall see, this capacity to make sense of trauma is at the core of a positive psychology of the human experience. But there is more.

Most professional concern with trauma has focused on single dramatic incidents, events that overturn reality for a few moments or a few hours, but which then are replaced with "things are back to normal." This is the stuff of 9/11 or tornadoes or being raped or witnessing a fatal shooting, *if* terrorism, powerful storms, sexual assault, and lethal violence are not part of the fabric of your day-to-day reality, *if* these events are disruptions of what is normal for you, what is good and safe.

If all this is true, then the experience of a single incident of acute trauma in an otherwise good life is likely to yield to short-term rest and therapy, a "therapy of reassurance" that through some combination of professional intervention and the goodness of everyday life brings a traumatized persons feelings and thoughts back into normal focus. This may be why research shows that writing about a traumatic event, particularly if that writing includes an effort to explain it and the response of someone who reads your account and comments, leads to improvements in both how people feel (subjective well-being) and how healthy their bodies are (e.g., better immune system function) [16].

Of course, the actual experiences of trauma victims differ. While some 80% do "get over it," some 20% do not, perhaps because their trauma experience was especially horrific (a vicious sexual assault, for example). But overall, the outlook for people experiencing single incidents of trauma in an otherwise positive life is very good.

My professional experiences in the world – in war zones, in refugee camps, in inner city neighborhoods, in abusive families – have led me to focus on the other kind of trauma, the experience of trauma that is repeated and persistent [17]. This is chronic trauma, when "normal" is the problem, not the solution. Chronic traumatic danger imposes a requirement for what we might call "developmental adjustment," in the sense that it demands a reorganizing of one's very understanding of life over time and not just a relatively short period of recalibration.

According to the influential theories of developmental psychologist Jean Piaget, our ideas about the world reflect the interaction of two processes [18]. The first is assimilation, when we are able to fit new experiences into our existing ideas. For example, once a child has the concept (or what Piaget called a "scheme") of dogs as four-legged furry creatures, the child can recognize various breeds of dogs; Labs, Poodles, German Shepherds, and Boxers are all examples of the concept of dog. But when a child comes across an animal that both is a dog and does not fit the requirements of the concept – perhaps by being too big, too small, too hairy, or not hairy enough – the child must change or adapt the concept of "dog" to fit the new information. It may even be necessary to add new concepts – for example, four-legged furry animals that are not dogs at all, but rather sheep, horses, or cows. This second process is called accommodation.

All this applies not just to the everyday concepts that we learn to make sense of the everyday world but also to how we come to understand the world when it comes to extraordinary experiences like trauma. When faced with trauma – particularly chronic trauma – we must undertake developmental adjustments that result from our inability to assimilate traumatic experiences into existing schema (conceptual frameworks), but rather demand that we accommodate – modify our concepts of how the world works or add whole new concepts of reality.

By definition (e.g., the APA definition), trauma is outside our normal "schema" or conceptual frameworks. Thus, traumatic experiences require us to alter existing concepts to permit the new experiential information to be integrated. This involves accommodation (using Piaget's terms). In the case of chronic danger, individuals (and groups) must accommodate their psychic realities so that they allow for the processing of life's atrocities. Put simply, they must adopt a view of the world that includes the reality of horror, violence, injustice, and vulnerability. From a Piagetian perspective, they have only their own emotional and intellectual resources to bring to bear on this task [19]. This increases the odds that how they accommodate to trauma will produce values and patterns of behavior that are not optimal either from the individual's perspective or from the perspective of the larger society.

This description reminds me why I have long found the Russian Lev Vygotsky's model of development [9] more satisfying than Piaget's explanation, since it provides additional dimensions to our efforts to make sense of and deal with trauma, one that more readily links to positive psychology, one that is more complete. By focusing on the intrinsically social nature of development, this approach highlights the role of "teachers" in mediating experience – whether it be the experience of learning about dogs or dealing with trauma, and this in turn increases the role of social and intellectual resources in dealing with trauma.

The key is Vygotsky's concept of the "Zone of Proximal Development," which posits that people are capable of one level of functioning on their own, but a higher level of functioning in relationship with the "teacher," who guides the "learner" toward enhanced development by offering responses that are emotionally validating and developmentally challenging. In a sense, the Vygotskian teacher aids in the process of accommodation, guiding it toward more sophisticated, adaptive, and "higher" concepts, schemas, and ways of thinking. In so doing, of course, this teacher can be the bridge between the base negative experiences of trauma and the higher experiences that are the focal point of positive psychology. This, it turns out, is one of the most important positive aspects of trauma and its aftermath, the opportunity to make a better world from the fractured ruins of the old, pretrauma world one knows.

How do human accommodations to traumatic events manifest themselves? Without effective "teaching" (in the Vygotskian sense), they are likely to include persistent posttraumatic stress syndrome, alterations of personality toward the self-defeating, value shifts toward the antisocial, and major changes in patterns of behavior that contribute to difficulties in the key relationships of normal life [19]. Chronic traumatic danger demands that those affected rewrite their stories, and redirect their behavior. These accommodations are likely to be especially pronounced when that danger derives from the violent overthrow of day-to-day social reality, when communities are substantially altered, when displacement occurs, and when individuals lose important members of their families and social networks.

For example, in the case of those exposed to the chronic horrors of Pol Pot's Khmer Rouge regime in Cambodia in the 1970s in which a third of the population was killed or starved and worked to death, 50% of youth studied exhibited persistent symptoms of PTSD 8 years after exposure [20]. According to psychiatrist Bessel van der Kolk, explosive outbursts of anger, flashbacks, nightmares, hypervigilance, psychic numbing, constriction of affect, impaired social functioning, and a feeling that one has lost control over one's life are all characteristic of traumatized people, particularly those who have not been "taught" to find alternative, positive meanings in their lives [21].

No single variable can be isolated as the leading cause of the damage that is so common among those living in situations of chronic trauma such as war zones (be they due to political violence – such as that due to conventional war or insurgency – or civilian community violence – is linked to gang activity). Rather, it is the interplay of several social and developmental influences that dictates the course and severity of the individual's maladaptation. Some do better than others; some even thrive, while others deteriorate. There are many factors that contribute to the range of outcomes. This, I think is because of what people are able to do and what help they have in doing it when they learn what I have called the Three Dark Secrets of Trauma [17].

The first of these three Secrets is that despite the comforting belief that we are physically strong, the fact of the matter is that the human body can be maimed or destroyed by acts of physical violence. Images of graphic violence demonstrate the reality of this. I call this *Snowden's Secret* after a character in Joseph Heller's 1961 novel "Catch 22," who is grievously wounded during a World War II mission on an American military aircraft. Hit by antiaircraft fire, airman Snowden appears to have suffered only a minor injury when first approached by fellow crewman Yossarian. However, when Snowden complains of feeling cold, Yossarian opens the young man's flak jacket, at which point Snowden's insides spill out onto the floor. This reveals Snowden's Secret: that the human body, which appears so strong and durable, is actually just a fragile bag filled with gooey stuff and lumps, suspended on a brittle skeleton that is no match for steel. People can learn this secret from their visual exposure to car crashes, shootings, and terrorist attacks, and it is one of the principal sources of trauma for them.

The second Dark Secret is that the social fabric is as vulnerable as the physical body, that despite all their power, institutions and authority figures cannot necessarily keep you safe when an enemy wishes you harm. Experiences in which parents, teachers, and other adults are present but unable to protect children effectively reveal this to children – and by extension adults as well. I call it *Dantrell's Secret* in commemoration of a little boy in Chicago who, in 1992, was walked to school by his mother [22]. When they arrived, teachers stood on the steps of the school, and a police car was positioned at the street corner. Nonetheless, as 7-year-old Dantrell Davis walked the 75 ft from his mother to his teacher, he was shot in the head and killed. Learning this secret can turn us away from the structures and values of social authority to fend for ourselves out of a sense of self-defensive adaptation, knowing now that society cannot protect you, that the social fabric of power and authority can be as fragile as the human body.

The third secret is *Milgram's Secret*, the knowledge that anything is possible when it comes to violence; there are no limits to human savagery. Stanley Milgram was the researcher who conducted what was certainly among the most controversial experiments ever conducted by an American psychologist [23]. He organized a study in which volunteers for an experiment on "memory" were positioned in front of a control board designed to allow them as "teacher" to administer electric shocks to an unseen "learner." The question underlying the study was, would the "teachers" administer what they knew were painful electric shocks to the "learner" if they were told it was their duty to do so. Before conducting the experiment Milgram surveyed people as to what they thought would happen in his experiment. Most people said that they thought "normal" people would refuse to inflict such torture and that only a few "crazy" sadists would do so. The results of the study were that although many participants were uncomfortable doing so, 65% of the "teachers" administered the torture – sometimes cursing the "learner" as they did so. This is Milgram's Secret, that comforting assumptions about what is and what is not possible all disintegrate in the face of the human capacity to commit violence when ordered to do so by an authority figure, particularly "for a good cause."

Milgram's Secret is coming to grips with the fact that any form of violence that can be imagined can be committed. True believers will fly planes into buildings at the cost of their own and thousands of other lives or will strap explosives on their bodies, walk into a school full of children and detonate the explosives, or will spread lethal chemical, biological, and radioactive toxins in the food and water of a community. Fathers and mothers will murder their children. Mobs will beat innocent students to death. Soldiers will burn down houses with their occupants inside. Whatever can be imagined can be done. Learning this secret can drive children and youth to emotional shutdown or hedonistic self-destruction, and adults to despair.

Historically, the origins of trauma have generally been limited to firsthand encounters with horror. But things have changed. The media technologies that emerged in the twentieth century added a new, unprecedented dimension to the psychology of terror by opening us to trauma induced by the vicarious experience of horror in full-spectrum imagery and sounds. One of the important elements of living in the current age is the growing recognition that modern mass media permit the conveying of traumatic experiences beyond those who are in-person witnesses, to the mass audience who are exposed to vivid visual and auditory representations of horror via videotaped records and through the simulations in video games, images that may be repeated over and over again.

This was observed in postoccupation Kuwait in the early 1990s, when videotapes of Iraqi atrocities were sufficient to elicit traumatic responses in children (who identified with the victims as their countrymen) [24]. And it is evident in the emerging body of research on the effects of violent video games, research that demonstrates their power to induce desensitization and increase violent fantasies, beliefs, and behavior, much the way that violence on television increases aggressive behavior in children [25].

Psychological connection to the immediate victims of horror is capable of transmitting trauma second hand. Add to this the fact of trauma research reporting that one of the elements in predicting whether or not a terrible event will produce long-lasting psychological symptoms of trauma is the degree of connection between the immediate victim and the second hand victim [26]. This finding resonates with a study of adult first responders who dealt with the carnage of a terrible bus accident, a study which reported that personal acquaintance with disaster victims is the most potent influence on whether those affected will exhibit stress reactions in response to a catastrophe [27].

This emergent definition of trauma and the role of second hand victimization via exposure to visual and auditory images of people with whom one has a psychological connection provide the first step in understanding how we react to war, family violence, and criminal assault in the community, as well as the "non-violent" trauma that occurs when children fall out of windows, drown in pools, lakes, and oceans, and when adults are killed in plane and car crashes.

One of the keys to understanding the dynamics of chronic trauma is to discriminate between the experience of trauma as "immunizing" vs. "sensitizing." Immunization is the process by which a person develops resistance to an "infectious agent" as the result of being exposed to something that is derived from or similar to that infectious agent. It allows the individual's immune system to prevent future illness when it subsequently encounters the infectious agent in question. We are all familiar with this model. You go to a clinic for an injection that prevents the flu in the future.

In the case of sensitizing, the first exposure leads not to immunity in the future, but to greater vulnerability. For example, consider what happens when children are hospitalized without parental presence. The psychological effects of one hospitalization on children are usually relatively minor [28]. It is the second and subsequent hospitalization that really causes problems, since rather than immunizing the child against separation anxiety, the first hospitalization sensitizes the child to future separations.

This is true in many aspects of human development, particularly those having to do with mental-health problems. Thus, for example, infants who are separated from their parents become more, not less, likely to have problems with attachment if they experience disruptions of parenting in the future. If an infant forms a strong attachment bond, the child is prepared to bond anew if transferred to a new parental figure [28]. But an infant who has already been subject to deprivation of the parent figure is a candidate for serious emotional problems if the second placement becomes a third and a fourth.

One model involves habituation, "getting used to" the disruptive event. The other model involves "kindling." Kindling means that repeated exposure results in the need for less and less exposure to cause an effect. Depression seems to work like this, for example. It usually takes a major negative life event to precipitate a first depressive period. But it takes less negative stimulation to set off a second, and still less to set off a third, just as once a fire has been burning in a stove, it takes less and less kindling to reignite the fire because the coals endure. In the case of "kindling depression," the brain begins to adapt to the process of repeated stress in a way that makes it more and more vulnerable to arousal that leads downward when challenging stimuli arrive [29].

So which is it in the case of trauma, immunization or sensitization? The preponderance of the evidence tells us that the answer is sensitization, but with a twist. In one sense, the sensitization model is clear in the research on the effects of chronic trauma. "Prior experience of trauma" pops up repeatedly when researchers ask which individuals are more likely to be exhibiting distress 6 or 12 months after a potentially traumatic event [26].

The twist is that one of the common consequences of chronic trauma often has the effect of making us *seem* unaffected by future traumas. Soldiers who have seen repeated combat often speak of "the thousand yard stare," to convey the cold look and flat affect that combat-weary veterans exhibit as a manifestation of acute stress reaction, part of the spectrum of responses captured by the symptoms associated with human reactions to trauma.

People with psychopathic personalities are stress-resistant because they do not experience the same degree of arousal in the face of threat that others do. How they get to this point is a matter of debate in the psychiatric community, with most subscribing to the idea that some people are born with neurological deficits that deprive them of the capacity to feel empathy and make positive human connections, but recognize that early experiences of severe psychological trauma can stimulate this neurological condition [30].

Whatever its origins, people with psychopathy do not have difficulty violating moral prohibitions with regard to killing human beings because they have no attachment to morality. Insofar as people with psychopathic personalities are hostile, emotionally impoverished, and detached, they do not become symptomatic in the face of trauma [30].

This finding would suggest that the individuals best able to survive functionally are those who have the least to lose morally and psychologically. In psychiatrist James Gilligan's terms, such people are already emotionally and spiritually "dead," and thus experience no fear or inhibition [31]. I don't know if I can accept the idea that their souls are dead or just deeply asleep, but in any case psychopaths view the world as having neither emotional barriers nor moral terrain. My own interviews of men incarcerated for murder and other acts of severe violence expand this view [17]. Some of the most violent youths construct elaborate defense mechanisms against anxiety, fear, and abandonment; these defense mechanisms culminate in the persona of the cold-blooded "gangster."

I see this often when I visit prisons as an expert witness to interview young men standing trial for murder. They often seem so cool and unaffected by what they have done, what has been done to them, and what they face in the future. But are they? Of course, there are human beings who come prewired for coldness, for emotional disconnection. Theirs are the ranks from which psychopaths come, but most traumatized and violent youth are not psychopaths.

How do "normal" soldiers, whether on the battlefield or the urban war zone, cope with repeated trauma? Until the point of breakdown they usually adopt a guise of numbness, coolness, and detachment. They do this whether they are military personnel in the national or insurgent army, or "soldiers" on the mean streets of violent neighborhoods. That's why the young men I see in court are so cool. Mostly they are not psychopaths (although some are). Mostly they are chronic trauma cases that have not yet reached the point of collapse [17].

So where does their trauma go, if not into the kind of overt disturbance and upset that is so common for first-time trauma victims in the immediate aftermath of their horrible experience? It goes inside, in the form of nightmares. It goes into the abuse of substances as a form of "self-medicating." It gets displaced into rage that diverts energy from sadness. It goes into the way their brain functions when aroused. It gets attached to fears that deflect attention from the primary fear. If we look for it we can find it in many places that at first glance seem like psychological red herrings (e.g., self-mutilation).

But this vulnerability is not the whole story, and it is only the beginning of the positive story about trauma, the story of getting to the other side of it. Some individuals who are not psychopaths demonstrate what has been termed "hardiness" in response to trauma, and this hardiness is the bridge to an approach to trauma grounded in positive psychology. For example, research by psychologist George Bonnanno [32] finds that soldiers who are rated high on this "hardiness" scale before they go off to war are less likely to suffer PTSD or serious depression when they go through combat. And, as noted earlier, research conducted by James Pennebaker shows that writing about trauma mobilizes this resilient hardiness [16].

Some resist the effects of traumatic experiences by developing unrealistically positive views of themselves, by repressing memories of the events to avoid confronting them, and by practicing positive emotions to displace sadness, grief, and anger. As Seligman notes in his review of the positive psychology research, in moderation, all of these may contribute to successful coping [33]. Seeing the glass as half full even if it is two thirds empty is a good strategy for preserving happiness and avoiding depression.

But hardiness seems to be so promising because it is more than simply refusing to confront traumatic experiences through self-delusion or repression. Rather, it is a matter of coping with adversity through positive strength, and as we shall see, it may open the door to understanding the dramatically *positive* experiences of life that stand in contrast to the negative effects of trauma. It is resilience built on the human capacity for finding meaning in life.

What are the elements of hardiness? [32] One is commitment rather than alienation. People who do not withdraw from life show greater resistance to the effects of experiencing traumatic events. In the face of the war or community violence or personal tragedy, one person says, "No matter what happens I still believe there is goodness in the world," while a second responds with, "I think all you can do is get as far away as you can and just forget about it."

A second element of hardiness is feeling in control, rather than feeling powerless. Particularly in Western cultures like our own, people place a high value on feeling powerful and in control, and psychological terms like "agency" and "effectance" speak to this [34]. It is understandable that if people feel totally out of control they are more likely to succumb to the psychological and philosophical effects of traumatic events. One person responds, "There are things I can do to stay safe," while another says, "I am completely at the mercy of the bad things in the world; there's nothing I can do about it."

A third element of hardiness is seeing the world in terms of challenge rather than threat. One person says, "We can find ways to make things more peaceful and I can be a part of those efforts," while another says, "All I feel is fear; fear that it will happen again and there is nothing I can do about it." Building upon these findings, psychologist Salvatore Maddi and his colleagues have developed a training program to enhance hardiness (the "HardiTraining Program") [32]. Its aim is to increase individual resilience in the face of life's bad things, in the face of trauma.

It's not all this simple, of course. We must be careful not to assume that people who are coping well with trauma in their day-to-day activities ("functional resilience") are necessarily at peace inside ("existential resilience") [9]. Some traumatized people who are very competent and successful on the outside are tormented on the inside. I have a friend who is spectacularly successful as a child psychologist, but whose inner life is tormented, and his intimate relationships often fractured. Any truly positive psychology must go beyond day-to-day functional resilience to consider the core inner psychological virtues of "thriving," "happiness," and "fulfillment." The key is to find ways to harness the human capacity for imagination to reprocess traumatic challenge into inspiration.

Related to this point is the fact that it is not enough to look at the effects of trauma in the short run. Some people maintain functional resilience for long periods – perhaps throughout their adult lives – while falling prey to existential despair later. A study of Dutch resistance fighters who were involved in the struggle against the occupying Nazi forces during World War II revealed that eventually all of them showed some effects of their traumatic experiences, although in some cases it was not until decades later [21] !

I have watched the television series "Band of Brothers" several times, and each time I force myself to listen to the painful first-person accounts of the soldiers recorded 40 years after World War II ended. It seems clear that "peace" was hard to come by and hard to sustain after going to war as they did. Some speak of how they held it all together as young soldiers, but as middle-aged men struggled to make peace with what they had seen, heard, and done. Trauma changes you forever. But it may take a long time for that change to become apparent.

When it comes to children, there are special issues and resources that contribute to resilience. Children look to key adults in their lives for cues and clues about what to make of powerful events that come to them via the mass media, and even directly from their observation of events in their immediate environment. This is one of the most important influences parents and teachers have on the children they care for and educate. The child's understanding of the world is very concrete. For a child, the most powerful question is "how is my world?" It is my house, my parents, my sisters, my brothers, my grandmother, my grandfather, my aunts, my uncles, my cousins, my toys, my pets. If that much remains intact, the child is rich in the most important ways in which a child can be.

This is not a matter of children being selfish, so much as it is the way children think: concretely. In fact, they can extend their caring to other beings, but it is mostly a matter of them making an emotional connection with those beings first so that they are added to the list of "my" attachments. For example, many children connect emo tionally with animals, so it should come as no surprise that surveys done during the Gulf War in 1991, revealed that the most upsetting media image for many young children was that of the water birds of Kuwait drowning in a sea of oil (caused by the efforts of the fleeing Iraqi forces to sabotage the Kuwaiti oil fields) [9].

In perhaps the earliest research on the topic of how children cope with living in a war zone, Anna Freud reported on children in World War II [35]. She found that if parents could maintain day-to-day care routines and project high morale, their children had a foundation of basic trust from which to build as they sought to cope with the stresses of war time life around them.

Perhaps the most important resource in building resilience in the face of trauma is forgiveness. Indeed, Seligman points to research by Everett Worthington and others [36] demonstrating the value of forgiveness – e.g., better overall health, and better cardiovascular health in particular. He writes, "forgiving transforms bitterness into neutrality or even into positively tinged memories, and so makes much greater life satisfaction possible" (p. 77). The bigger the trauma, the more difficult it is to forgive, but the more important to do so. This brings us to one of the foundations for forgiveness, namely, compassion.

The Dalai Lama teaches that compassion is more than a feeling dependent upon the sympathetic character of the other [37]. It is the ability to remain fixed on caring for the other person regardless of what that person does, not just out of sympathy for the other person. It is also from the recognition that it is best for ourselves to live in a state of compassion rather than hatred, in part because it stimulates forgiveness. One of the Dalai Lama's most important lessons is this: true compassion is not just an emotional response, but a firm commitment founded on reason.

It is easy to feel hatred for our enemies and sympathy for the victims of violence – particularly when we ourselves are those victims. It may seem paradoxical to some, but compassion provides a foundation for healing much more so than it does simply holding a grudge and seeking revenge. These approaches only fix us in our trauma, and usually sustain a cycle of violence. I know that is why I have sought to forgive the obstetrician whose callousness compounded the pain when my daughter Joanna was struggling to be born. Letting go of him was important in freeing myself to be there for my daughter.

This compassionate response does not mean simply ignoring evil, violence, and sin. It means that even in the face of human behavior that is evil, violent, and to our sensibilities sinful, we still care for the offender, even as we seek to control that person's dangerous behavior and protect ourselves and the community. Indeed the crucial concept for those who seek to live by compassion is to hold the sources of their trauma within "the circle of caring."

In the film "Seven Years in Tibet," a European friend of the young Dali Lama begins work on a building. He arranges for workmen to dig a trench as the start of creating a foundation. As they begin work monks approach them and ask them to stop the digging because they are killing the worms. For them, the circle of caring includes even the lowly worm. None of God's creatures is excluded, and each creature deserves care and concern. And the Dalai Lama has lived up to his ideals in the decades since he fled from Tibet to escape Chinese oppression by holding his Chinese "enemies" within his circle of compassionate caring. As he himself acknowledges, this has been difficult, but at the same time a prerequisite for his own positive psychology to flourish.

The perpetrators of trauma linked to war, family violence, and criminal assault in the community typically are caught up in their own scenarios of revenge and retaliation. Often they have experienced personal suffering or family loss, or historical victimization, and are seeking a way to give meaning to that suffering through acts of violent revenge rather than compassion and forgiveness. Mostly, they are individuals who are offered a political or ideological interpretation for their situation by their leaders, or cultural support for abusive treatment of children and spouses, or incentives provided by criminal leaders.

Sometimes these leaders are pathologically calculating and cold in their exploitation of their followers. Sometimes these leaders themselves are plotting revenge for what they have experienced as victims of oppression. For them the acts they commit are not "unprovoked assaults," but rather are their own, sometimes warped, version of "bringing the perpetrators to justice." We must not fear this understanding. We must not reject those who ask for understanding. We must remember the wisdom that teaches, "if you want peace work for justice." And remember what Gandhi taught when he said, "you must be the change you wish to see in the world."

Dehumanization is the real enemy. Each individual has a story to tell, a human story. The great psychiatrist Harry Stack Sullivan wrote that "people are more simply human than otherwise" [38]. What he meant is that we must always seek a human explanation for the way people behave, no matter how irrational, demented, or monstrous it seems at first glance. This is an excruciatingly difficult task when the behavior in question is war, family violence, and criminal assault in the community. But it is essential that we do so for very practical as well as very noble reasons.

In all these cases it is a matter of strength of character and wisdom to choose forgiveness where it is forbidden or denigrated or equated with weakness. I have seen this firsthand. Not long after my book *Lost Boys* came out, I received a call from a woman who mysteriously asked to meet with me in private to discuss a dilemma with which she was wrestling, a dilemma related to youth violence, the topic of my book. We met in a local restaurant, where she told me the nature of her problem. It seems her favorite niece had been murdered by the girl's boy friend, who was apprehended and sentenced to a long prison term for the crime.

This woman had been devastated by the death of her niece and could not understand what to make of the boy's violence. But unlike all the other members of her family, she wanted to understand, so she secretly visited the boy in prison, and having met him began to visit him regularly. She told me that if the rest of her family knew what she was doing, they would disown her. Her dilemma was that once she met the boy she felt compassion for him and was moving in the direction of forgiving him. Understanding him – his inner torments and his capture by the worst of masculine violence – was a threat to her rage, but she felt alone in her compassion and feared being actively rejected by her family if that compassion led her to forgiveness. This was all true, but nonetheless she knew that her best chance for finding enduring happiness – what Seligman would call "authentic" happiness – in her life lay in forgiving this boy. I felt that she was correct in her assessment, and counseled her to proceed cautiously but determinedly down that path (even if it meant living a double life with respect to her family), which she did.

Ultimately her bravery and wisdom transformed her life in positive ways she could not have anticipated, as has confronting violent boys and men with compassion transformed mine, if only "second hand" as an emotionally engaged professional, not a direct victim. Coming from the other side of the fence, so to speak, several times a year I receive letters from men and boys who are incarcerated for violent crimes who, like the woman whose daughter was murdered, have read *Lost Boys* and found in it a voice that speaks to them about compassion and forgiveness. Some of them have undergone a profound spiritual transformation as part and parcel of fully owning their crimes and simultaneously seeing the roots of that crime in the way they themselves were victimized and traumatized by others, earlier in their lives.

The lesson here is that the experience of injustice and trauma offers spiritual opportunities just as it offers moral challenges [9]. How we respond goes a long way in determining whether we will emerge with a positive psychology of trauma. What influences whether we seize and profit spiritually from these experiences, or simply allow them to feed the dark side of our human selves, our needs to be powerful, in control, and angry?

One person who has illuminated the choice we face is psychotherapist Dave Richo [39]. Richo has looked closely and with unblinking eyes at how the needs of our egos can push us away from the spiritual opportunities posed by trauma toward the darkness that comes with revenge, anger, and retaliation. He writes, "Injustice leads to rightful indignation, attempts to repair the abuse, and grief about the loss. Grief is scary mainly because it seems to equal powerlessness. Its alternative, revenge, is resistance to grief, since it substitutes retribution for sadness. It grants a false sense of power because it is power over others, not power for resolving unfairness or transforming human beings" (p. 90) [39].

How does this translate in the world? Richo sees one of its manifestations in the application of the death penalty. "Capital punishment is an example of a historically legitimized form of revenge. It is rationalized as deterrence. Our wounded ego engages the state to assure we can get even and not have to grieve so ardently or be so much at the mercy of life's conditions. Once we let go of ego, love gains precedence in our hearts and we cannot be satisfied with punishment. We want the transformation of the offender, restitution to us or the community, or the offenders' heartfelt restoration to humanity" [39].

But what are we called to do in response to those who hurt and despise us? Richo defines it as "utter reconcilability." By that he means that we must not allow our hurt egos and our dark sides to use the opportunity presented by traumatic events to liberate and validate our rage. Rather, we must seek out the greater wisdom of making peace with all and everyone. Every religious tradition and every spiritual path offers guidance on this matter. The Christian recipe for divesting ourselves of ego violence and retaliation is to be found in the Sermon on the Mount. There we find the unpalatable recommendations that we turn the other cheek, bless those who hurt us, love those who hate us. In short, reverse every automatic reaction of ego. Richo sees this same impulse in other religious traditions. In many ways, Buddhism is founded on just such paradoxes, namely, that finding authentic happiness lies not in feeding the ego but in starving it, a theme to which I return later, in Chap. 5.

Compassionate spirituality reflects a willingness and ability to be maximally inclusive in defining the "circle of caring," the domain in which people are entitled to our highest moral concern [9]. As one spiritual teacher puts it "To be 'spiritual' means to know, and to live according to the knowledge, that there is more to life than meets the eye" [40]. Compassion is the commitment to care for "the other" despite fear, anger, and disappointment. Compassionate spirituality is always suspect in our society, as it is in many others.

Promoting resilience refers to ways in which we can enhance our ability to deal with trauma constructively and successfully. A crucial component of this resilience is confidence in the future – hope. In the television age in which we live, trauma is brought into our lives in historically unprecedented ways, and this trauma threatens our foundations for hope and future orientation, and in extreme cases replaces future orientation with "terminal thinking." But even when it comes to terminal thinking, there is human potential to be considered, a positive psychological perspective to be applied, as the following story indicates.

A professional colleague of mine has a psychotherapy practice in Washington, DC. She tells the story that one morning on her way to work she received a call on her cell phone from a friend who had just been to see her doctor and had been informed that she had a fast-acting cancer and would be dead in six months. Her friend told my colleague that she was on her way to the bank to withdraw her life savings, and was then going to buy herself a sports car and a mink coat. "After all," she said, "what am I saving for?" Later that morning, when my colleague arrived at her office she watched out the window as her first client arrived, a young drug dealer from one of the most violent neighborhoods in the city. He was wearing a mink coat and driving a sports car. A light bulb went off in her head, and my colleague realized her client and her friend had the same "problem" of terminal thinking, one induced by a cancer death sentence, the other by the death sentence of living with intense and probable deadly violence as a drug dealer on a daily basis.

But this is not the end of this story, a story that I have told repeatedly in my lectures on trauma and resilience. A year later, I was the keynote speaker at a conference in upstate New York on prospects for positive development among high-risk youth. Before my talk I was chatting with the conference's organizer, a 60-something woman who I had met 30 years earlier at a summer camp, which she attended with her children, and where I had been a counselor. I had seen her occasionally since that summer camp experience, but not for the past five years.

When I innocently asked her how things were going, she replied that she had terminal cancer, and was not expected to live through the year. But she was not wearing a fur coat and she was not driving a sports car. She was organizing a conference on youth development. She was living out her last months as she had lived most of her life, devoted to helping others, fulfilling her commitment to a better world, smiling. She had attained something beautiful in her life. Something positive in her psychology sustained her, so she had no need for the delusions of material possessions in an impossible effort at self-comforting. Having chosen the deeper positive path, she was comforted and she was authentically happy. She had met the challenge of trauma successfully, and crossed over to the other side, where she could be a great "teacher" to her children, her friends, her colleagues, and many people other people, including me.

Was she deluding herself? No, I don't think so. As Daniel Gilbert has shown [15], the key is to find ways to harness the human capacity for imagination to reprocess trauma into inspiration. In this process we can look to developmental psychologist Lev Vygotsky's insight on the role of "teachers" in development [19]. These are the people who help us move from where we are to where we could be, to traverse the "zone of proximal development" to arrive at a point where we can see bigger and deeper meaning to life events, the point at which we can see the good in the bad, and perhaps even see the good in the terrible. My friend had done just that. I thank her for bringing a bit of beauty into the world that so desperately needs every bit of spiritual beauty that anyone of us can uncover.

References

1. http://www.jstor.org/pss/20409912.
2. Shion, P. and Quinn, L. (1994) Living arrangements of children. Children and Divorce, 4, 1ff.
3. Child drownings. http://www.poseidon-tech.com/us/statistics.html – figure adjusted for 1958 child population.
4. http://www.airdisaster.com/special/special-aa191.shtml.
5. http://www-fars.nhtsa.dot.gov/Main/index.aspx.
6. http://findarticles.com/p/articles/mi_m1370/is_v19/ai_4004412/.
7. http://academic.evergreen.edu/g/grossmaz/interventions.html.
8. http://www.aolnews.com/world/article/record-number-of-journalists-murdered/19412693.
9. Garbarino, J. (2008) Children and the dark side of human experience: Confronting global realities and rethinking child development. New York: Springer.
10. Ambrose, S. (2001) Band of brothers. New York: Simon and Schuster.
11. Grossman, D. (2009) On killing: The psychological cost of learning to kill in war and society. Boston: Back Bay Books.
12. Herman, J. (1997) Trauma and recovery. New York: Basic Books.
13. http://www.emdr-therapy.com/.
14. http://www.psych.org/mainmenu/research/dsmiv/dsmivtr.aspx.
15. Gilbert, D. (2007) Stumbling on happiness. New York: Vintage.
16. Pennebaker, J. (1997) Opening up: The healing power of expressing emotions. New York: The Guildford Press.
17. Garbarino, J. (1999) Lost boys. New York: Free Press.
18. Piaget, J. (2001) The psychology of intelligence. New York: Rutledge.
19. Vygotsky, L. and Kozulin, A. (1986) Thought and language. Cambridge, MA: MIT Press.
20. Sack, W.H., Clarke, G., Him, C., Dickason, D., Goff, B., Lanham, K., Kinzie, J.D. (1993) A 6-year follow-up study of Cambodian refugee adolescents traumatized as children. Journal of the American Academy of Child and Adolescent Psychiatry, 32, 431–437.
21. Van der Kolk, B., MacFarlane, A., Weisaeth, L. (2006) Traumatic stress: The effects of overwhelming experience on mind, body and society. New York: Guildford.
22. http://www.chicagotribune.com/news/politics/chi-chicagodays-dantrelldavis-story,0,6132262.story.
23. Milgram, S. (2009) Obedience to authority: An experimental view. New York: Harper.
24. Nader, K. and Pynoos, R. (1983) The children of Kuwait after the Gulf crisis. In: L. Leavitt and N. Fox (eds). The psychological effects of war on children. Hillsdale, NJ: Earlbaum. Pp. 181–195.
25. Bushman, B.J. and Anderson, C.A. (2001) Media violence and the American public: Scientific facts versus media misinformation. American Psychologist, 56, 477–489.
26. Eth, S. and Pynoos, R. (1985) Post-traumatic stress disorder in children. Washington, DC: American Psychiatric Publishing.
27. Terr, L. (1992) Too scared to cry: Psychic trauma in childhood. New York: Basic Books.
28. Rutter, M. (1989) Developmental pathways and resilience. Journal of Child Psychology and Psychiatry, 30, 23–51.
29. Kramer, P. (1997) Listening to prozac. New York: Penguin.

30. Hare, R. (1999) Without conscience: The disturbing world of the psychopaths among us. New York: Guildford Press.
31. Gilligan, J. (1997) Violence: Reflections on a national epidemic. New York: Vintage.
32. Bonanno, G. (2004) Loss, trauma, and human resilience: Have we underestimated the human capacity to thrive after extremely adverse events? American Psychologist, 59, 20-28.
33. Seligman, M. (2004) Authentic happiness. New York: Free Press.
34. White, R. (1959) Motivation reconsidered: the concept of competence. Psychological Review, 66, 297–333.
35. Freud, A. and Burlingham, D. (1943) War and children. London: Greenwood Press.
36. Worthington, E. (2003) Forgiving and reconciling. Isla Vista, CA: IV Books.
37. Dalai Lama (2009) The art of happiness: A handbook for living. New York: Penguin.
38. Evans, F.B. (1996) Harry Stack Sullivan: interpersonal theory and psychotherapy. New York: Routledge.
39. Richo, D. (1999) Shadow dance. Boston: Shambhala Publishing.
40. McBrien, R. (2008) The church: The evolution of Catholicism. New York: HarperOne.

Chapter 4
What Is the Opposite of Trauma? The Positive Power of Transformational Grace

I began this book with a commitment to bring to bear the concepts of positive psychology to my own life in the hope of shedding light on the human condition. In the previous chapter I delved into the *worst* of the issues in what might be called "negative psychology," namely, trauma, but sought to show how meeting this challenge with positive psychology *can* lead to growth and development, at least for some people, some of the time. But what then is the *best* of issues for positive psychology? I think it is to be found in asking, "what is the opposite of trauma?" But there is a prior question, namely, "how would I know?" And that is where I must begin, with the challenging of knowing.

After many years of professional and personal struggle to know things about human nature, human behavior, and human development, I have come to the conclusion that there are not one but three principal paths to knowing: "science and humanities," "subjective human studies," and "soul searching." A complete understanding of a human life and the human condition requires all three.

Let me give an example of how these three ways of knowing coexist in the real world, an example that mirrors the issues we face in life as a whole. Consider the process of playing a game – perhaps a game of my favorite sport, baseball. The outcome of the game hinges on the skill of the players as well as random variations in success (and the premise of fair and competent umpires, of course). So where do the three ways of knowing come into the game?

The science of the game hinges on the fact that the link between the skill of the players and the outcome of the game is neither fixed nor completely random; it is, as most things in science are, a matter of probabilities, of odds. On average, the team with the best players will win more often than not. The most skilled players will reach base safely more often. The best pitchers will strike out more batters than less talented pitchers. This is particularly true of baseball, where even the most successful of players rarely get a hit more than 30% of the time, and where numbers play an important role in documenting the progressive history of games (and the best teams in professional baseball win little more than 60% of their games).

The new science of "chaos theory" expands upon this basic principle by revealing that physical and social reality is composed of interlocking systems, systems that interact with each other in often subtle and very complex ways. Thus, while it is

J. Garbarino, *The Positive Psychology of Personal Transformation:*
Leveraging Resilience for Life Change, DOI 10.1007/978-1-4419-7744-1_4,
© Springer Science+Business Media, LLC 2011

often impossible to predict how any individual event will progress, when enough events occur, they will reveal underlying patterns. The unpredictability of individual events subject to the subtle interplay of complex forces has come to be known as "the Butterfly Effect," after the fact that the actions of a single butterfly flapping its wings in the Amazon River valley could set off a chain of events that would lead eventually to a hurricane in the Atlantic Ocean.

In this, the case of the butterfly mirrors human life in many important aspects. For example, the odds that a human being will live to be 80 years old are known at birth based upon gender, social class, time, and place. The odds are particularly good if you are born in the twenty-first century in a middle-class family living in an affluent First-World country like the USA where overall life expectancy is 77 years, and rather poor if you are a born in a destitute family living in a village in a Third-World country like Bangladesh, where life expectancy is 59 [1]. Beyond these general probabilities in the USA, there is the added effect of gender on the odds, with the average woman living 6 years longer than the average man. But odds only apply to large numbers of multiple events and never completely account for outcome: some men live longer than some women, just as weak hitters sometimes hit home runs and strong hitters sometimes go hitless for several games in a row.

To return to the sports metaphor, from the perspective of "subjective human studies perspective," a baseball game (like each of our lives) is about each contestant's specific experience and what it means to that individual. Some players are stronger, more coordinated, and more knowledgeable than others, but whether or not this translates into a hit or a winning game is not known in advance, nor is the meaning that players attach to their success and failure.

The key biographical dimension of the game lies in the fact that the significance of playing and whether or not you win the game depends upon who you are as an individual. For me as a fan, for example, it matters a great deal whether "my team" (the New York Yankees) wins or loses. While I can appreciate the skill of an opposing pitcher who strikes out "my" team or the opposing batter who hits a towering home run against "my" pitcher *in the abstract*, what matters to me emotionally is that it is Yankee pitchers who dominate and Yankee hitters who hit home runs.

Why is this? Some of it derives from the fact that I grew up in New York City (although I had friends who were fans of the Brooklyn Dodgers or the New York Giants before both teams moved to California in 1958, many of whom shifted their allegiance to the New York Mets when they were founded in 1962). But the principal reason I grew up a Yankee fan and remain one to this day is that my father was a devout Yankee fan. Going to a Yankee game or even watching one on television evokes my father for me, the memories I treasure of attending Yankee games with him when I was a child, and the love I had and have for him, though he died more than 20 years ago.

Playing baseball itself has strong biographical links to my father: he played catch with me for hours so that I might learn the basic skills of the game. And, he sometimes watched me play the game. This was a source of emotional satisfaction for me, win or lose, because it was a bond between us (and he accepted me, win or lose). All those feelings flood over me when I watch a neighbor playing catch with his son across the street from our house.

But what does baseball mean for children observed by parents who seek their own gratification in their child's athletic performance, for a child of low self-esteem or for one with intense emotional investment in being a winner. For these individuals, the stakes in each game, indeed in each at bat, are high. When I was a kid playing baseball, I knew such kids – and was sad for them when I saw the pressure their fathers imposed on them to perform. And for another child (not so competitive as I) the result of a game or an at bat may be of trivial importance, in comparison with the pleasure of playing the game and being part of a team. It all depends on who you are and what baseball means to you. For me, one of the most intense personal meanings of "playing baseball" is tied to the first time I started a game as a high-school varsity player in right field, and dropped a line drive to allow the winning run to score in the last inning. Like many "traumatic" memories it is available to me still, in vivid sensory detail more than four decades later. Today when I watch the Yankees play and an opposing player hits a sinking line drive to right field, my body tenses up in expectation of that error I made when I was 17 years old.

The knowledge that comes from human studies may extend to the subjective meaning of the baseball game in general, however (the place at which social science and human studies intersect). Some 3 decades ago, one of my professors at Cornell University – Edward Devereux – produced a documentary film simply entitled "Two Ball Games" [2]. In it, children are observed playing baseball in two contexts. One is an informal, "sandlot" game with no adult involvement or supervision; the other is a formal Little League game that is coached, refereed, and judged by adults (coaches, umpires, and parents).

In fact, some of the same children participated in each game. Devereux's short film follows the progress of each game without any narration, from start to finish, illuminating how the process and meaning of this sporting event is very different for the children in the two settings. The film culminates with the losing pitcher in the Little League game crying in frustration on the bench, while the informal game ends with two of the players riding off on the bicycles asking, "who won?" with little regard for the outcome.

Here too, the game mirrors human life on Earth. Each of us has a personal story. These stories are particular to our "luck" from day to day and year to year, our talents and abilities and how our environment welcomes or rejects them, and how we respond to these events to create our emergent stories.

For example, some people in both the affluent First World and the destitute Third World defy the statistical odds of their situation: some Americans die in the first year of life; some Bangladeshis live to be 90. What is more, among both children and 90-year olds in every society, there are variations in the perceived quality and meaning of their lives. Some poor kids experience a story of happy, content meaningfulness, while some rich kids tell a story of sadness, despair, and nihilism. Whatever it is, each individual's story is a unique expression of how he or she encounters and experiences life, even as science documents the odds of this happening or not happening in each group.

What about soul searching? From a deep perspective, the baseball game is at best an amusing and entertaining diversion. Trophies or other prizes to be won are minor matters. While in general, life may be more comfortable with success on the playing field (the average salary of players who reach the Major Leagues is about $3 million!), soul searching reveals that if the process of obtaining or having any form of worldly success distracts from enlightenment and love, it is a dangerous delusion.

It's only a game, after all, *as is everything material that does not nourish spiritual life.* Once again, this mirrors human life in general. From the perspective of spirit, how long you live is not the issue, but always "how well." I thought of this in October 2002, when I was asked to deliver a talk at a church in Virginia at the time that the "Beltway Sniper" was at large – shooting people at random in the area of the church.

I recall the conference organizers' concerns that attendance would be down because of people's fears of going out in public and thus exposing themselves to the shooter. I remember the palpable anxiety as my host and his family exited their minivan and walked from the parking lot to the church building. As I stood at the pulpit, I spoke of the irony of this situation. Certainly one of the core beliefs of Christianity is that you must always be ready for death by living a life of faith. Jesus spoke of this, saying "I am the resurrection and the life. Those who believe in me, even though they die, will live." (John 11:25).

It is a testament to the difficulty of living completely in congruence with our spiritual beliefs that the many Christians attending the conference found it impossible to live as their faith instructed them to do. Living the life guided by the spirit is easy in the abstract, but awfully difficult in the reality of day-to-day life.

The issue is always how you live the time you have. In the Fall of 2005, two deaths occurred in my social world within the space of one week's time. The first was my 88-year-old mentor, psychologist Urie Bronfenbrenner, who died after a life of enormous professional accomplishment and family proliferation (five children, 16 grandchildren and two great grandchildren). The second was a 10-year-old boy in my church who died after living most of his life with cancer. To all who knew him, the little boy's life was completely fulfilled spiritually, even while it was grievously abbreviated as a biography and was a physical catastrophe in scientific, objective terms.

In the eternal world of the spirit, our time on Earth is a very minor matter, made significant only by virtue of the fact that it affects our opportunities to engage the universe and progress toward enlightenment. By all accounts, the little boy with cancer lived a very "spiritually efficient" life in the sense that he achieved a rare level of consciousness and closeness to God in the few years of life on Earth available to him. No one would invite cancer into the life of child just to create the opportunity for spiritual growth and consciousness, of course, but there is no denying that ultimately it is the spiritual "accomplishments" of living that matter most. The film "My Sister's Keeper" in 2009 portrayed this message beautifully, as a 15-year-old girl dying of cancer teaches her family important lessons about achieving peace with the end of life, whenever it comes.

Having made the three forms of knowing concrete through an example, let me return to each in a more elaborated way, as a preparation for exploring how each affects the way we seek to understand the opposite of trauma. Science and humanities are the domain of academics. Here we find the efforts of scientists and humanists.

The former (both physical and social scientists) seek to demonstrate the objective empirical realities of human behavior. The latter look for patterns in culture and history by analyzing literature and other human documents.

The goal of the scientists is to document empirical patterns, statistical relationships, and predictive and verifiable hypotheses concerning the objective features of human development. This is what scientific psychology – positive, neutral, and negative – is all about. The humanists seek to tease out of documents larger patterns of meaning, themes in history, literature, philosophy, and art. This is what the "history of psychology" attempts to do, and what many nonscientific psychologists attempt in their work.

Whether they are scientists or humanists, this is the predominant discourse of those who work in academic psychology. It is the world of "on average" and "in general" and "on the whole" and "most" and "few" and "many." Both science and humanities have at their core a set of rules and principles to govern the pursuit of knowledge and its communication to others. In this sense both are "objective." This is not to say that biases don't creep into the process. They do. But the intellectual beauty of science and humanities is that there are well-established tactics and strategies for exposing and disposing of these infringements upon the fundamental commitment to objectivity when they are detected, for "falsifiability."

Perhaps it is a digression of sorts to pursue this matter and perhaps I expose a bias that I inherited from Urie Bronfenbrenner when I say this, but it does seem that one domain of psychology that may be an exception to this is psychoanalysis. Here it seems that "falsifiability" is largely unobtainable (because every exception to every rule can be and, in my experience often is, dismissed as "reaction formation" or some other way out of confronting the fact of a proposition being false). On more than one occasion Urie said to me of psychoanalysis "never has so much intelligence and energy been devoted to explaining things that have never been demonstrated to exist." Said like the scientist and humanist he was, and more than a little true, I think.

I read a couple of books by Sigmund Freud when I was in high school – and would often disappear into the local library on a summer afternoon as part of my campaign to educate myself beyond what a suburban secondary school in the mid 1960s might provide. By the time I came to graduate school, I had absorbed Urie's critique of psychoanalysis, and perhaps had taken it too far – to the point of dismissing it entirely. It was not until 1985, when I became president of Erikson Institute, an independent graduate school focusing on child development that my world view expanded. Erikson Institute had been found by three early childhood educators with a psychoanalytical bent and it offered me an education in the value of this perspective – at least as a source of intelligent, creative, and insightful hypotheses, if not as a methodology for testing these hypotheses empirically. It made a difference in how I have looked at human development since. But I digress.

At the core of empirical studies is the hypothesis – the "supposition about fact." Formulating hypotheses and testing them is the bread and butter of empirical studies, whether they be science or humanities. One of the principal strengths of empirical studies is that it is open to hypotheses from any source. The model of the DNA double helix came to researcher James Watson as a flash of inspiration (fueled by a lot of hard work by him and others) [3]. Others have generated hypotheses on the basis for painstaking incremental research – with each study a next step in a long progress of studies each adding a small variation on the previous ones. Still others have generated hypotheses from anecdotal personal experiences – like psychologists Eleanor and James Gibson who developed the hypothesis of the "visual cliff" [4] on a family trip to the Grand Canyon, when they disagreed about whether their young children would naturally know to stay back from the edge of the canyon or would need to learn this ability (the results of their research showed that this ability was largely innate).

Empirical studies require a radical openness to validation and falsification that runs against the human grain in many ways because humans are prone to detect patterns where they don't exist, overgeneralize coincidences, and stick to their guns even as counter evidence accumulates. Many fields of human endeavor exemplify the process by which hypothesis is confused with proof. Let's consider reincarnation as an example. The hypothesis that people have multiple lives, that they are reincarnated, is an appealing and powerful one. It would help to explain child prodigies like Mozart: how did he play and compose so well at such a young age? Answer: He practiced in previous lives and was able to carry that knowledge and skill into the life he began on January 27, 1756. How to explain why people often report dreams in which they are living in an earlier time period as someone else? Answer: They are recalling memories of experiences brought from previous lives. How did a young child in Tibet named Lhamo Dondrub correctly identify items that belonged to the 13th Dalai Lama, who had died in 1933 – 2 years before the child was born? Answer: The child was the 14th reincarnation.

I must say that I like the idea of reincarnation. But liking the idea does not mean that it is proven. Setting aside the many possible conceptual and technical issues in reincarnation (many of which have been addressed by Tibetan Buddhism and other systems that rely on it as a foundation), there is one issue that vexes me, and until it is resolved makes reincarnation "only" a hypothesis, and perhaps a dubious hypothesis at that.

Historical demographers tell us that due to rapid population growth in the twentieth century, the nearly seven billion people currently alive on the planet represent about *half the people who have ever lived* on Earth [4]. This means that there have only been enough human lives in the past that each one of us today could only have had one human life before this one, and if current demographic trends continue, soon there will not be enough left in the past for all of us to have had one. That's OK if reincarnation has only happened once for all of us (with some of us coming back from a long time ago and others, indeed most, from times quite recent). But for any of us to have had more than one past life as a human being, someone else must have had none. With many accounts of reincarnation speaking of multiple past lives (I know people who claim ten or more) a corresponding number of current residents on Earth must either be "new souls" or have come from somewhere else in time and space, and their accounts of having lived before on Earth are mistaken perceptions.

Personally, I like the "new souls" explanation, since it fits nicely with my observation that most of us don't seem to have the faintest idea what we are doing here when it comes to the big picture. It does require me to believe that those who do claim to have had multiple past lives on this planet reflect some combination of them being "special" and that it is a coincidence that everyone who comes to a past life specialist just happens to be one of those special people. Of course, the alternative is that most people who believe that they or others have lived past lives are deluding themselves or fabricating for the benefit of others.

I am open to all solutions to this problem so long as they deal with it as a real problem for the empirical study of reincarnation. They don't, however, as far as I can tell. Amazon.com lists more than a thousand books dealing with past lives and reincarnation. I haven't read many of them, but in the ones that I have looked at I don't find this issues dealt with. My wife and I have Tibetan friends (and are the god parents for a Tibetan child), so we have regular contact with Tibetan Buddhist monks. One night we hosted a small dinner party that included four monks, one of whom was a particularly distinguished teacher (Geshe). I asked him my question about numbers and got nowhere. A follow-up session a couple of years later did lead to the admission by a couple of our Tibetan friends that most people do not have past human lives, but "earned" coming back in this life as a human because of their success in past lives as nonhumans (animals and insects). That certainly makes some sense.

The Dalai Lama's answer is that there are many alternative worlds in which past lives take place: that there are other dimensions coexisting with ours and that this is where the other bodies are to provide homes for the reincarnated spirits who have the multiple lives. This might be considered the "Star Trek" explanation, and I am open to this hypothesis (as a confirmed fan of "Star Trek"), even though it does mean that most of the reports of past lives on Earth are understandably mistaken. But what it is not is proof. It is not what empirical studies is all about, the testing of hypotheses. I consider the question open pending further explanation and study.

But while science and the humanities map the large-scale psychological, sociological, biological, cultural, and demographic terrain of human development, this alone does not lead us to the end of the journey when it comes to knowing. Set within this conception of life is the individual experience of being human, which inescapably leads us to a second methodology, the study of subjectivity in what some scholars have called human studies.

"Human studies," as the term was used by psychologist Bert Cohler [5], is the study of the unique meaning that individuals recognize in themselves, and the processes and strategies for communicating that meaning to others, albeit inadequately. There are an enormous number of specific influences on any single individual human being, influences with interact and accumulate to produce very different end results. Therefore, no two human beings share exactly the same life pathway, and no two of us have exactly the same autobiography. No matter how much I am like other blue-eyed, bald, Caucasian college professors born in 1947 in New York City of English mothers and Italian-American fathers, no two of us are exactly the same – inside or out. My life story is mine alone in very special ways.

There are general commonalities, to be sure, and these are the object of study by science and humanities – for example, in a branch of psychology called "life span development" [6]. And there are points of perfect intersection between separate lives, the points at which two individuals recognize that despite the myriad of differences that differentiate them as people, there is a point of complete correspondence, an experience that may lead them to define each other as "soul mates." Claire and I have this, despite our many discontinuities, disagreements, and incompatibilities. She likes to quote the lyric of a Donny Hathaway song ("A Song for You": "I love you in a place where there's no space or time"). I like it too. Of course, actually living together in this space and time is always a challenge!

Subjective human studies recognizes that each individual life is unique in the experiencing of it. It asks us to try to walk miles in the shoes of another human being. But even as it asks us to adopt this strategy for feeling what the other feels – empathy – it recognizes that whatever we learn will be intrinsically and inevitably incomplete and approximate. This differentiates human studies from science and humanities, where precision rules.

Subjective human studies demands that we allow room for a process that moves beyond the constraints of a purely academic focus on objectivity and verification. It demands that we allow for subjective information to become a valid vehicle for understanding human experience. Human studies focuses on the narrative accounts of subjective experience, on life stories, and on autobiography.

It's about discovering and assessing the meaning of human experience as it is lived and understood by a specific individual. It's about human beings in their singularity as represented through the stories these human beings employ to make sense of themselves as individuals (and as members of groups). Human studies is the documentation of identity: it is you telling the story of your life, and me telling the story of mine. It's the study of autobiography.

Human studies seeks to illuminate subjectivity, while acknowledging that any such effort can only be partial, no matter how long we work at it and how smart we are. It recognizes that no matter how good the story, how poignant and evocative the language of that story, and how diligent the listener's efforts, there is always loss of validity from the teller of the story to the listener. What we learn from the creating and telling of our life stories advances our understanding of the human experience. But it too is incomplete.

In other words, empathy is never complete. In human studies you can never know exactly what I am experiencing, unlike in science where, when I say the temperature of this liquid is 45°F you can know exactly what that means and exactly replicate my data (even though if you say that 45° feels cold and I agree, we cannot be sure that we mean the same thing). Philosophers of science have called this phenomenon of you knowing what I know (and I knowing what you know) "inter-subjective transmissibility" [7].

All human communication is ultimately imperfect. Thus, intersubjective transmissibility is always and inevitably partial and incomplete. But even were it to be complete, it would not be the whole human story because human beings are more than the story of moving their bodies around on the planet Earth. Human beings are spiritual beings having a physical experience on the planet, and this requires yet another kind of knowing.

This third form of human study is soul searching. Here the goal is to make and sustain contact with spiritual realities beyond the facts of physical experience, and even the individual's subjective account. And, like science and humanities, there is a defining methodology to soul searching.

What is this method? It is contemplation, meditation, and prayer. It is what Zen Buddhists like Thich Nhat Hanh call "mindfulness," the practice of paying attention to reality "in the present moment" [8]. It is to sit quietly for a long time and focus your attention – perhaps through observing your breathing or through meditative prayer. The evidence is clear that if you follow this methodology you will reach approximately the same conclusions as others before you have. Some time after I wrote these words, I read Karen Armstrong's book *The Spiral Staircase* [9] and her conclusion after she conducted a deep comparative study of the world's major religious thinkers and wrote: "Working in isolation from one another, and often in a state of deadly hostility, they had come up with remarkably similar conclusions. This unanimity seemed to suggest that they were onto something real about the human condition" (p. 289). Amen to that!

In this sense, then, science and humanities share with soul searching the goal of documenting and illuminating common realities, while human studies seeks to document and illuminate particular realities. In the case of soul searching, these common and "objective" conclusions find expression in statements such as these three: "there is more to life than the material experience of it" and "love is the fundamental imperative of the universe" and "peace comes from caring without attachment to self and to outcome." To quote Karen Armstrong again, "The one and only test of a valid religious idea, doctrinal statement, spiritual experience, or devotional practice was that it must lead directly to practical compassion. If your understanding of the divine made you kinder, more empathetic, and impelled you to express this sympathy in concrete acts of living kindness, this was a good theology. But if your notion of God made you unkind, belligerent, cruel or self-righteous, or if it led you to kill in Gods' name, it was bad theology" (p. 293) [9].

As in the case with science and humanities, the particulars of what exactly this means in day to day life are sometimes somewhat ambiguous and open to dispute. In Buddhism, for example, the basic data of soul searching are represented as The Four Noble Truths: life means suffering, the origin of suffering is attachment, the cessation of suffering is attainable, and the path to cessation of suffering lies in a practice that avoids extremes, neither hedonism nor asceticism. In Christianity, the basic data of soul searching are represented by the Sermon on the Mount and the other hopeful teachings of Jesus. In science, it is represented by positive psychology.

From this perspective, religion is the intellectual and social infrastructure created to house and promote these three basic "findings." Thus, each religion is its own "take" on these primary data – part of what my Jesuit friends mean by the expression "finding God in everything and everyone," and why they have been so interested in finding spiritual truths and realities in every culture they encounter. What is more, some individuals discover these data without the benefits (or obstacles) of any specific religion so long as they follow "the method," while others get so caught up in the institutions and verbiage of religions that they never come close to the spiritual realities that lie under them.

Apply the method and you reach the three basic data of soul searching, just as if you embrace the methodology of science and direct your attention to human biology you come to the conclusion that the current form of human bodies is the product of evolution – despite the claims of "creationism" or "intelligent design." Similarly, whether you are the Christians St. Ignatius of Loyola or Mother Theresa, or the Buddhists Thich Nhat Hanh or the Dali Lama, the common method leads to the same essential mission in life, although how you express these truths and what implications you draw for day-to-day living in the specific cultural and historical context of your life may vary. And, each tradition develops complex and detailed expositions on the implications of the basic data of soul searching, which being human are always incomplete, frequently misleading, and sometimes dead wrong.

Some Native-American cultures speak of "soul traveling" as a way to integrate the experience of body/mind/brain/soul. Christian, Jewish, and Muslim mystics see the path in prayer. Buddhists and Hindus speak of insight meditation. This approach starts from the reality of human beings as spiritual beings having a physical experience, and proceeds from there. Does anything in human experience really mean anything beyond what individuals, groups, and cultures say it means? Is there anything more than psychology, biology, sociology, and anthropology on the one hand, and history and literature on the other? Without soul searching, the answer is "no." With soul searching the answer is "yes."

If we do not recognize the spiritual realities underlying the literary realities of narrative accounts and the statistical descriptions of empirical realities of the social and physical sciences, there is only one empirical reality – "You are born. You live. You die." – and only two basic narrative accounts: "I am born. I have a nice day. Then I die." or "I am born. My life sucks. Then I die."

Only soul searching can expand these stories by integrating them into the eternal realities of spirituality. The two traditions with which I am most familiar – Buddhism and Christianity – offer elaborate worldviews that transcend the experience of conventional life and place the individual in the realm of the timeless, where oneness with the universe becomes "obvious." You can't go there without this spiritual practice (but limiting yourself to the theology and practice of conventional religion may not take you there either because these are derivative of soul searching not soul searching itself).

And what of the question with which I began this discussion, "what is the opposite of trauma?" What is the answer? If trauma is fundamentally "something negative from which you never recover," the simultaneous experience of overwhelming negative arousal and overwhelming negative cognitions, then its opposite must be "something wonderful you never can lose," the simultaneous experiencing of overwhelming positive arousal and overwhelming positive cognitions. What might we call this? I think we can call it "transformational grace," the realization of all that soul searching teaches us about human life in ways that changes how and why you live. *When all is said and done, perhaps nothing is of equal importance to a complete positive psychology.*

What does it mean to experience overwhelming positive arousal? For many people the first answer that comes to mind is sexual orgasm. While men and women differ in describing the particulars of orgasm (and most certainly report differences in how likely it is to result from everyday sexual intercourse), most of us would be tempted to cite the pleasure that comes from consensual sex as a candidate for being "the opposite of trauma." Nearly a century ago, psychoanalyst Wilhelm Reich [10] proposed that "orgastic potency" was the key well-being psychologically (and physically, for that matter). But is it truly the opposite of trauma, this overwhelming positive arousal?

Sex certainly can offer overwhelming positive arousal – just as it can offer overwhelming negative arousal when things are not right (e.g., in cases of rape). But the fact that it *can* offer overwhelming positive arousal is not enough by itself to qualify it as fully the opposite of trauma, however. The second element – overwhelming positive cognitions – is as necessary to qualify as transformational grace as are overwhelming *negative* cognitions to justify the diagnosis of trauma. The arousal must *mean* something.

An experience of overwhelming negative arousal without meaningful consequences is not trauma; it is a bad scare, a fright. I sat in a movie theater recently watching the previews for the coming attractions. The movie I was waiting to see was one that was clearly marketed for the "youth" audience, since the trailers shown were mostly for some variety of modern horror films – in which there are vivid images of truly horrible events (gory decapitations, bloody eviscerations, that sort of thing). But the young people sitting behind me in the theater did not find the images traumatic. For one thing, they are so familiar with contemporary vivid special effects that they found the horror at best momentarily arousing (while I and the other older members of the audience were authentically horrified).

But after a second, they (and indeed most of us older viewers) knew that these images and the films from which they came did not *mean* anything; they were just entertainment. Thus, the worst that could happen to these young people is that they would get a good fright from the movies. Of course, some children watching the same scenes could be traumatized by these images because they have less capacity to appreciate them as entertainment and more as potentially real (and they are less desensitized to the horror of the images than the older kids in the audience). Indeed, psychologist Dorothy Kanter's research has documented long-term effects of traumatic movie images presented to children – e.g., the 1975 movie "Jaws" [11].

Having disposed of positive arousal without positive cognitions, what about the experience of overwhelming positive cognitions without the arousal? This too can be important, but it is not transformational grace. Perhaps the best word for it would be an inspiring idea. For example, according to the best estimates of modern astronomers, there are thought to be about 100 billion (100,000,000,000) stars in our galaxy, and about 80 billion galaxies in the universe, which means there are about 1,000,000,000,000,000,000,000 stars in the universe [12].

When I think about that and the fact that each day life on Earth depends upon the influence of just one of those stars, I am cognitively overwhelmed, positively overwhelmed because it puts my life – indeed all human lives, all six billion of us – in perspective. I find this idea transformative in the sense that it reorganizes my whole relationship to the universe. But I think about it and then I go back to business as usual. Why? Because it is only a cognition, and without the overwhelming arousal it remains a limited, though inspiring, thought.

How might it become an experience of transformational grace? It would require that I have the sensory input to go along with the thought. As it happens, I had precisely that one day in the O'Hare Airport in Chicago. I was standing on a moving walkway en route to the United Airlines terminal. On the wall was a series of photos provided by the Adler Planetarium, taken from the Hubble Telescope, orbiting the earth 350 miles above us. Each documented an array of galaxies – hundreds and thousands of them. These pictures reached me on a deep emotional level. Photo after photo provided visual imagery to bring to life in my senses what I *knew* to be true before: my physical being is less than an infinitesimal speck in the universe. But the coupling of the cognition with the arousal made it the source of transformational grace, if only for an intense moment, but a moment that may linger a life time if I pay attention, something I can renew any time I want by going to the Hubble telescope Web site [13].

It should be clear by now that the parallel when it comes to the opposite of trauma is that for sex or any other overwhelming positive arousal to be a meaningful experience, perhaps a spiritual experience, or even something that constitutes transformational grace, the arousal must be coupled with overwhelming positive cognitions. It must demonstrate something positive that transcends normal reality (in the way that trauma's three dark secrets demonstrate something about the dark side of human experience). Are there Three *Bright* Secrets of Transformational Grace to parallel the Three *Dark* Secrets of Trauma I spoke of in the previous chapter? I think so. The Three Bright Secrets of Transformational Grace are these:

Benedict's Secret: Mellen-Thomas Benedict "died" from a brain tumor in 1982, returning to life an hour and a half later [14]. He provided a detailed account of his "near death experience," and has spent the years since making sense of his experience and its implications for how he lives his life and communicating its implications to others (http://www.mellen-thomas.com). The core insight he returned with is this: physical experience is just the beginning of human reality. Human beings *are* spiritual beings having a physical experience on this planet, and encounters with the magnificence and beauty of the natural and social worlds can reveal this truth, even if this encounter only comes in death.

The Good Samaritan's Secret: The Parable of the Good Samaritan appears in the biblical book of Luke (Chap. 10: verses 25–37) and has come to represent a compelling message about compassion in the face of adverse social conventions and self-doubts. The Samaritan helps a victimized stranger, who belongs to a group with whom Samaritans share an abiding hostility. The message is this: the human capacity for goodness is amazing, and it offers a path to Heaven. Encounters with altruism and service can inspire an appreciation for the wondrous positive potential of human life that elevates us, and in so doing stimulate transformational grace.

Buddha's Secret: After nearly 10 years of searching, the Indian prince Siddhartha realized that enlightenment is possible. He spent the rest of his time on Earth exploring and communicating the practices and beliefs that flowed from this insight. Buddha's Secret is that Heaven is here in every present moment for those train themselves to know how to see and feel it. Knowing this pushes aside conventional fears, concerns, and suffering, and puts our divine opportunities center stage.

One of the important distinctions within our understanding of transformational grace parallels the distinction within trauma studies of "acute" vs. "chronic." Recall that in the case of trauma, acute, single incidents pose different challenges to the psyche than do chronic, multiple threats. The former can readily be dealt with by a therapy of reassurance, and are unlikely to lead to widespread long-term consequences. Chronic trauma, in contrast, requires developmental adaptation and is more likely to lead to widespread long-term consequences, consequences that can spread beyond individuals to infuse culture and social institutions. I believe the same distinction applies to transformational grace.

What are the acute incidents? They are the moments of insight that come from mind-blowing encounters. In the movie "The Bucket List," the characters played by Jack Nicholson and Morgan Freeman make a list of "things to do before you die." Having both been diagnosed with terminal cancers, this is a topic of great urgency for them, and using Nicholson's character's great wealth to finance their activities, they set off to check items off the list. First on the list is "Witness something truly majestic." For this they travel to the Himalayan Mountains. The amazing vistas they encounter fulfill the mission.

This kind of transcendent encounter with the magnificence of nature exemplifies acute transformational grace. I have had these experiences, as have most of us in one way or another in the course of a lifetime. For me they include a hike in the "Grand Canyon of Hawaii" on the island of Kuai. These breathtaking experiences of nature qualify as acute incidents of transformational grace. But they can also include encounters with the glory of human creations as well. One example for me was my first encounter with Venice, Italy: on a sunny summer day Claire and I emerged from the train station, and there before us was the Grand Canal in all its glory. It took my breath away and changed the way I looked at the world – at least for a short period of time. I can recall the experience, but only in muted form, a faded reincarnation of that incredibly vivid moment, that at the time I vowed I would never let go of!

These "human creations" can also include amazing acts of selflessness, courage, or compassion. While traveling in Vietnam with a group of colleagues in June 2008, I witnessed such an act when the one American combat veteran in our group met up with some Viet Cong veterans who had served in the same time and place as he in the late 1960s. Watching their encounter, these once fierce enemies exchanging hugs and smiles as comrades, was as spectacular as the Grand Canal in Venice – and, I must say, equally ephemeral in its permanent effect on my consciousness.

Like acute trauma, the likelihood that acute incidents of transformational grace will result in long lasting let alone permanent change is small. Some people really do reorient and alter their lives in response to such a moment, but most slip back into ordinary normality once "things get back to normal," just as they do when the have experienced an acute trauma. It may take months – in either case – but this is the sad truth. It has long been recognized in the study of religious conversion experiences, sensitivity groups, ecotravel experiences, outdoor therapy programs, and all the other wonderful short-term encounters with beauty, truth, and wonder that litter the cultural landscape. For example, a colleague of mine on the Vietnam trip was so moved by our visit to an orphanage that he vowed to give up his life in Chicago and return to devote himself to the welfare of the children. I saw him on campus months later, and regular reality had retaken hold of him.

I have been to many of the world's truly majestic places, among them Lake Atitlan in Guatemala and Lake Como in Italy. Both are stupendous in their beauty, and do indeed inspire awe. Encountering them – certainly encountering them for the first time – truly produced an experience of transformational grace, but only a momentary one. These encounters did not change my life. That required the very ordinary lake around which I walk Hope and Dharma.

This little lake is literally "nothing to write home about." It is small – perhaps a mile in length and at its widest a quarter of a mile wide. It is shallow. It is surrounded by marsh in many places and by low hills in others. It is really just the man-made result of a small dam built during the 1930s by the New Deal's Civilian Conservation Corps that stopped the unimpeded flow of a stream, and created a run of the mill state park. But it is in the detailed, ongoing encounter with this lake, its surroundings, and its animal residents that chronic transformational grace is to be found. Even as insensitive as I am, I am often moved by the subtleties of inspiration at this lake.

Although I am not a poet, one morning on a late summer's day even I was moved to write a poem to capture the essence of that day's walk around the lake with Hope and Dharma, a poem in the form of a Haiku (a Japanese unrhymed form that usually focuses on nature or the change of seasons, and contains only 17 syllables arranged in three lines):

Hot forest, August.
Ten red leaves spill the secret:
Fall is coming soon.

On another occasion I was mesmerized by a circle of the bright morning sunlight intensely reflected off the lake through an opening in the trees. These are the building blocks of chronic transformational grace, and because they are embedded in a "practice" of morning walks, they are different from the acute experiences that come from *visiting* majestic vistas.

It is the difference between visiting majestic lakes and living with any lake, between a weekend sensitivity group and sustaining an altered relationship with self and others, between a revival meeting and a meditative or prayerful practice, between attending a workshop on joy and living a life informed by the activities and virtues that Seligman's research [15] demonstrates are reliably related to building up a trait of positivity (rather than just slipping in and out of a state of happiness), the virtues, the acts of service, the attention to positive thoughts, the being embedded in sustaining relationships, the flow of good work.

On one of my trips to the Middle East, I had the opportunity to visit the site at the north end of the Sea of Galilee (as Christians tend to call it, of Lake Kinneret as it known by Israelis) where Jesus offered what has come to be known as The Sermon on the Mount. I was traveling with a group, and someone had brought a Bible and read the text of the section called "The Beatitudes" as it is presented in The Gospel of Matthew. As the warm breeze on that sunny day flowed over us gently, the text's words were truly transformative as each message of blessing flowed over us like the gentle breeze. Blessed are the poor of spirit, they that mourn, the meek, the hungry, the merciful, the pure in heart, the peacemakers, and the persecuted. Hearing the words at the site of their origin infused them with greater meaning than they ever had for me before.

The simplicity of this as a practical religious experience made of it a kind of Zen Christian experience – to complement the Zen Buddhist experiences I have had over the years. But I can't live at the north end of the Sea of Galilee, so I find the direct experience I need in contemplative prayer in my home church. Perhaps I should locate my religious life as a Quaker, with their simple stripped down practice of prayer, but I find the nearly empty noon Catholic Mass in the glorious Madonna del la Strada church on the Loyola University campus offers the same spiritual opportunity, as does the meditation room in our house.

Chronic transformational grace is, like its counterpart in chronic trauma, an alternative reality in which "normal" is the source of ongoing, even permanent positive change. In one sense, just as the therapy of reassurance is ineffective in treating chronic trauma, so the details of ordinary life are ineffective in destroying chronic transformational grace, or at least they can be if one has fully integrated the fruits of transformational grace into one's mind and heart.

Of course, few people are capable of such a complete integration that they are immune from the corrupting influences of ordinary life. Perhaps those who meditate "professionally" like the Dalai Lama or Thich Nhat Hanh are such individuals. I have read their books and observed them both firsthand, and I suspect they have so fully made transformational grace the essence of their being that they could spend a week watching reality shows like "Real Housewives of Hollywood" on television and doing a 9-5 boring clerical job, and yet still remain in a state of transformational grace. They would still even find a way to fit in their regular four hours of a day in meditation.

But even these highly evolved persons did not start from a position of transformational grace. They achieved it the old fashioned way: they earned it through a long process of meditation, study, and prayer that led to a shift in consciousness that is supported by a day-to-day practice of mindfulness. They have devoted their lives to soul searching. Thich Nhat Hanh writes: "Relief, peace, well-being, joy and better relations with others will be possible if we practice mindfulness in our everyday life. I am convinced that everybody can practice mindfulness, even politicians, political parties, even the Congress. This is a body that holds the responsibility for knowing the nation's situation well, and knowledge of this kind requires the practice of looking deeply. If our elected officials are not calm enough, do not have enough concentration, how can they see things deeply?" [16] (True Love, in the chapter titled "Everybody Should Practice Mindfulness").

What stands in the way of achieving transformational grace? There are the daily distractions of modern life, of course: television, video games, materialist vulgarity, physical sensations that capture our attention, fear, lust, and all the "isms" that divide and conquer us. But those who seek to live with transformational grace are united in identifying one paramount impediment: attachment to the self and the religion of ego, namely, narcissism in all its individual and collective forms, and to that we turn our attention next.

References

1. http://www.worldlifeexpectancy.com/.
2. http://www.css.washington.edu/emc/title/2981.
3. http://www.dnalc.org/search?fl=catalog:DNAi&.
4. http://www.wadsworth.com/psychology_d/templates/student_resources/0155060678_rathus/ps/ps05.html.
5. Cohler, B. (1991) The life story and the study of resilience and response to adversity. Journal of Narrative and Life History. 1, 169–200.
6. Santrock, J. (2008) Life span development. New York, NY: McGraw Hill.
7. Husserl, E. (1970) The crisis in European sciences and transcendental phenomenology. David Carr (trans.) Evanston, IL: Northwestern University.
8. Hanh, T.N. (1990) Peace is every step. New York, NY: Bantam.
9. Armstrong, K. (2005) The spiral staircase: My climb out of darkness. New York, NY: Anchor.
10. Reich, W. and Carfagno, V. (1986) The function of the orgasm. NY: Farrar, Straus, and Giroux.
11. Harrison, K. and Cantor, D. (1999) Tales from the screen: Enduring fright reactions to scary media. Media Psychology. 1, 97–116.
12. http://www.imagine.gsfc.nasa.gov/docs/ask_astro/answers/970115.html.
13. http://www.hubblesite.org/.
14. http://www.mellen-thomas.com.
15. Seligman, M. (2004) Authentic happiness: Using the new positive psychology to realize your potential for lasting fulfillment. New York, NY: Free Press.
16. Hanh, T.N. (2009) Happiness: Essential mindfulness practices. Berkely, CA: Parallex Press.

Chapter 5
Can There Ever Be Enough Me? Narcissism and the Positive Death of Self

Western, non-Buddhist psychology is all about self, and usually in a very positive way (with one major exception as we shall see). As a result, self-esteem and self-concept (and the lack of them) are topics of a great deal of psychological research and speculation in our psychological tradition. At the same time, the relationship of self to others is understood to be central to a healthy development of self. "Attachment" is considered one of the pillars of mental health (at least if it is "secure" rather than "anxious-ambivalent," "anxious-avoidant," or "disorganized"). Attachment theories start with a focus on the human tendency to seek closeness to another human being, with the result being the child feels secure when that person is present – and anxious when that person is not present [1]. It's a positive need, and meeting it creates positive spin-offs for a lifetime – positive psychology.

Secure attachment is considered the foundation for mental health and good relationships generally. Thus, "attachment disorder" is a serious pathology, expressed as "failure to form normal attachments," and there are therapies to deal with it. "Reactive Attachment Disorder" is an official psychiatric diagnosis that reflects profound problems with forming and sustaining positive attachments, starting in early childhood (and usually associated with grossly inadequate early care, the kind found in some terribly run orphanages and in neglectful and abusive families) [2].

In mainstream thought, the model for optimal human development is relatively simple: attachment is good, and nonattachment or nonsecure attachment is bad. The good comes in the form of an internal model of positive relationships that generalizes beyond parents to include other intimates, and from infancy across the life span [3]. The badness comes in some mixture of disturbed social relationships and disturbed self-concept that poisons all relationships, starting in childhood and continuing onward through adolescence into adulthood.

Positive psychology is certainly pro-attachment. Seligman's book has multiple references to "secure attachment," which is fitting given the overall focus on *positive* psychology. He writes, "Securely attached children grow up to out perform their peers in almost every way that has been tested, including persistence, problem solving, independence, exploration, and enthusiasm [4]." And "The bottom line is that by almost every criterion, securely attached people and secure romantic relationships do better." (p. 195) I agree with Seligman about the developmental

J. Garbarino, *The Positive Psychology of Personal Transformation:*
Leveraging Resilience for Life Change, DOI 10.1007/978-1-4419-7744-1_5,
© Springer Science+Business Media, LLC 2011

benefits of secure attachment in this conventional psychological sense – who couldn't? However, when viewed through the lens of Buddhism's Four Noble Truths, attachment beyond relationships in infancy and childhood is *the problem not the solution to the human condition*. And, although the scientific case may be closed with respect to the developmental benefits of attachment, the psychology of "self" is a different matter.

"Self" is itself a major preoccupation in psychology – always has been. Efforts to locate the self within the social environment have a long history as well [5]. One danger that astute observers of American culture and society return to over and over again is that the profound individualism of our culture will generate social estrangement and that this will cause us grief – individually and collectively. This theme has echoed across the decades, from William Webb's "parabola of individualism" [6] and David Riesman's *The Lonely Crowd* in 1950, [7] to Phillip Slater's *The Pursuit of Loneliness* in 1970 [8], and most recently Robert Putnam's *Bowling Alone* (2000) [9] and John Cacioppo and William Patrick's *Loneliness: Human Nature and the Need for Connection* (2008) [10].

In this tradition, Seligman speaks approvingly of a concept of self that is warmly embedded in positive relationships, evoking the Japanese concept of "amai" – "the sense of being cherished and the expectation of being loved that children raised correctly attain [4]" (p. 213). Reading this I was reminded of Martin Rotenberg's analysis of "Alienating Individualism and Reciprocal Individualism: A Cross-Cultural Conceptualization" in 1977 [11]. In it, he argued that because we define dependence as pathological and autonomy as healthy, we doom ourselves to a pervasive sense of estrangement and alienation, and offered amai as a healthy alternative. Consistent with its tradition of being the keeper of the flame for positive psychology pre-Seligman, Rotenberg's analysis was published in *The Journal of Humanistic Psychology*.

But much as some psychologists have validated a positive concept of dependence (or at least "interdependence") as a corrective to the corrosive and often toxic nature of individualism, this has not resolved the matter. Western psychology continues to struggle with the alienating inertia in our culture, an inertia born of individualism and a focus on an individualistic concept of self [12]. Others have gone so far as to pose a dimension of social connection as independent of self, permitting a fourfold scheme in which combinations of high and low self-concept coexist with combinations of high and low social orientation. As in most such "2×2 tables," the result is a series of types. Many have looked to one such effort in particular developed more than 40 years ago.

In a 1966 book entitled *The Duality of Human Existence*, David Bakan [13] proposed two dimensions for the self in the world: "agency" (referring to self-enhancement and self-assertion) and "communion" (referring to group participation and cooperation with others). As rendered by psychologist David Buss in 1970, Bakan's analysis sees it this way: The agenic person forms separations; the communal person creates unions. The agenic person isolates self from others; the communal person embeds the self in a collective. The agenic person exists for the self; the communal person provides for the group. Unmitigated agency, according to Bakan, propels both the individual and society toward destruction and death. (p. 556) [14]

"The mitigation of agency with communion, therefore, provides a proper goal of the individual throughout life." (p. 236) [13]. As so often is the case, some Aristotelian Golden Mean is offered as the healthy alternative to any extreme form.

Not much is written about three of the four extreme types in Bakan's system: low agency coupled with high communion, low agency coupled with low communion, and high agency coupled with high communion. The first might be called the "meek-embedded" (ineffectual, but prosocially oriented and connected). The second might be termed the "loner-loser" (powerless and disconnected). The third might be termed the "powerful do-gooder" (prosocial, but in the service of the self). It is the fourth combination, however, that receives the most attention.

Unmitigated agency might be called "too much self," and when it is coupled with a deficit of communion, it has a name in mainstream psychology: "narcissism." Like terms such as "trauma," narcissism has multiple definitions – some more evocative, others more precise. At the evocative end are emotionally loaded words such as "egotistical bastard" and "self-centered asshole." At the more precise and cooler end of the spectrum are "excessive self-love based on inflated self-image or ego, coupled with a lack of empathy for others." Whatever the words used, it represents a high level of agency (self-serving and self-promoting in the world) and a low level of communion (disconnected emotionally from the best interests of the world outside self).

What is narcissism about? The term itself derives from the Greek myth of Narcissus – a handsome young man who was punished for rejecting the advances of the nymph Echo by being forced to fall in love with his own reflection in a pool of water and spend the rest of his life pining away because he could not consummate his love, for himself. The modern manifestations reflect this myth in the sense that today's narcissists are so caught up in making themselves the center of attention that the needs of others, indeed the very psychological reality of these others in many cases, disappears from their consciousness. In its place are self-centered and usually manipulative efforts to retain a unidirectional flow of love and attention from the other to the self. In many accounts, and in keeping with the original myth, narcissists ultimately suffer themselves because by living a life of disconnection, they starve themselves of important psychological nutrients as they seek to sustain themselves on the unhealthy diet of solely self-validation.

Some of the best fleshing out of the negative impact of narcissism comes from the many books and Web sites written by people who have lived with – or tried to live with – narcissists, and have the emotional scars to show for it. It's easy to find evidence of this simply on the internet by searching for "narcissism jokes." The result is a series of Web sites that collectively provide a long list of "jokes" about narcissism, often bitter and sad jokes to be sure, but the message is clear.

Here are some particularly clever examples:

How many narcissists does it take to change a light bulb? One. He holds the bulb while the world revolves around him.

What do a narcissist and a sperm have in common? Both have about a one in three million chance of becoming a human being.

My husband and I divorced for religious reasons. He thought he was God and I didn't. (from http://www.drirene.com).

Then there are these, in which cleverness plays second fiddle to bitterness:

Why does a narcissist get upset or moody after having just spent lots of time in his/her own company? Well how would you feel just after having spent lots of time in the company of a narcissist?

Psychiatrist interviewing narcissist Psychiatrist: "What is your favorite Christmas carol?" Narcissist (with a straight face): "Hark the Herald Angels Sing About ME."

Why does a narcissist find it so difficult to empathize with others? Because he (or she) is always so busy empathizing with himself (or herself).

How do you get a narcissist to respect other peoples' preferences? You can dream! (from http://www.lisaescott.com/forum).

The standard tool used by mental-health professionals in diagnosing Narcissistic Personality Disorder [15] identifies a list of nine traits, possessing any five of which qualifies for this diagnosis:

- Grandiose sense of self-importance
- Preoccupation with fantasies of unlimited success, power, brilliance, beauty, or ideal love
- Belief that he or she is "special" and unique and can only be understood by, or should associate with, other special or high-status people (or institutions)
- Need for excessive admiration
- Sense of entitlement
- Takes advantage of others to achieve his or her own ends
- Lacks empathy
- Often envious of others or believes that others are envious of him or her
- Shows arrogant, haughty behaviors or attitudes

Naturally, this is but one end of a continuum [14]. At the extreme other end might we find some sort of pathological selflessness (assuming that selflessness can ever be thought of as pathological). As we shall see, the operative mechanism in functional narcissism is high self-esteem, so perhaps the pathological opposite of narcissism is a sense of profound worthlessness – like the man who gave away all his money and even donated vital organs to others because he did not think he could justify existing while others were dying [16].

There are "healthy" points on this continuum, of course. On the healthy side but on the selfless end might be extreme altruism and compassionate caring. One place where this plays out is in the donations of kidneys. According to a National Kidney Foundation survey, [17] about 25% of the respondents said they would be willing to donate to a stranger. As *New Yorker* journalist Larissa MacFarquhar [16] found out when she explored this issue, more than 7,000 people have signed up as potential donors in the first five years of operation of a commercial Web site (http://www.MatchingDonors.com) that connects them with people in need of a kidney transplant, and more than 600 have already gone through the surgery.

Their motives? They ranged from a highly evolved and self-aware altruism (like Kimberly Brown-Whale, a female Methodist minister-missionary who said

"If you're sitting around with a good kidney you're not using, why can't someone else have it.") to self-deprecating neediness (like Rob Smitty, who initially was attracted by the thought that he could sell his kidney for $250,000 but then when he found it was illegal to do so went ahead anyway, saying when he was jailed for nonpayment of child support, "I thought maybe the judge would cut me some slack – I donated a kidney, I can't be that bad – but it didn't happen that way.")

Consider the example of Paul Vandenbosch, a father of four, aged 54, who donated a kidney to a woman whom he did not know and has never met to save her from kidney failure, spare her the ordeal of dialysis, and help to restore her to health and a normal life. And, Melissa Stephens, who wrote about donating a kidney on her blog, "I have always felt loved, cared for, secure, content, inspired and grateful for the family I was given…and I want to give back some of the love I've received." Now that the medical procedure for donating a kidney is nearly risk-free, giving one kidney in this spirit seems prosocially heroic but still with a positive sense of self-worth to validate continuing to live oneself. Nonetheless, most donors report negative reactions from their family and friends to their gesture of giving. It seems most people see this act as pushing the envelope of "communion" too far [16].

Surely there is a healthy point on the selfless side of the continuum. But is there such a point on the narcissistic side? While severe narcissism is recognized as a personality disorder with terrible clinical implications, what some psychologists call "normal narcissism" is associated with positive mental health in mainstream psychological terms. In this view, self-esteem is the link between narcissism and psychological health in the sense that their reservoir of self-regard gives them a buffer against negative experience. Psychotherapist Wendy Behary has offered a compassionate analysis of the varieties of narcissism in her book *Disarming the Narcissist: Surviving and Thriving with the Self-Absorbed* [18]. Clinical psychologist Linda Martinez-Lewi focuses on the "high-level narcissist" and offers a much more harsh and much less compassionate view in her book *Freeing Yourself from the Narcissist in Your Life* [19].

Seligman [4] reports that people who think positively about their past and their future are happier – and live longer and healthier lives. One way to accomplish this is to believe in your worth as a person, your competence in dealing with the world, and having a sense that you are entitled to good things in life and therefore to see the past and the future through glasses that are at least somewhat rose-colored. Remember that, in Seligman's positive psychology, inaccurate positive perceptions generally lead to more happiness than accurate negative ones. With respect to the past, Seligman recommends, "satisfaction, contentment, fulfillment, pride, and serenity." For the future, he suggests "optimism, hope, faith, and trust." For the present: "joy, ecstasy, calm, zest, ebullience, pleasure, and (most importantly) flow." (p. 62) [4].

All of these could well be linked to positive self-concept. If you have a strong sense of Bakan's "agency," you could well feel positive about day-to-day life (since you have a lot of success in the world), positive about the past (since you have a record of achievement and acknowledgement), and positive about the future (since you trust that the world will continue to receive you and your efforts well).

The problems would arise if your agency was misplaced – in the sense that you really aren't as competent as you think you are – or unfairly judged – if people have biases and prejudices that distort their assessments of you, such as racism, sexism, homophobia ("heterosexism"), ageism, or any of other "isms" that unfairly lead to degradation and rejection where there should be acknowledgement and acceptance.

Studies by Constantine Sedikides and his colleagues [20] reported in the *Journal of Personality and Social Psychology* in 2004 focused on the mental health of young people who do not show the *extremes* of narcissism that would qualify them for a diagnosis of Narcissistic Personality Disorder. On the Narcissistic Personality Inventory (with a possible range from 0 to 40), the average scores in the groups studied were about 6, 16, 17, and 12 for four groups of undergraduate psychology students and 13 for a group of married couples in their 30s (with a range from 2 to 39 – an important point because to the degree that the NPI is used as a diagnostic tool for narcissism it focuses on scores above 35). The researchers found that so long as the tendency toward narcissism does not reach extremes, it is associated with a variety of positive mental-health outcomes: less daily sadness, anxiety, and depression, and a greater sense of well-being. These outcomes include a sense of marital well-being in couples – at least among the well-educated young people studied.

However, virtually all the effect of narcissism on psychological well-being was accounted for by the high self-esteem that these individuals demonstrated (the agenic dimension, in Bakan's terms). Take out the high self-esteem and the other aspects of narcissism (related to low communion and grandiosity) appear to be related to lower psychological health. Perhaps this is why the bottom line is a mixed picture for the narcissists themselves (particularly if their self-esteem becomes deflated) and frequently a long-term problem for the people who are in (or who at least *think* they are in) the narcissist's life.

Like most things, the utility of narcissism depends upon the context in which it occurs. Believing in themselves (even if unrealistically so) and having a good sense of how to present themselves when initiating contact or in superficial relationships, narcissists don't worry much or feel gloomy. In a society like ours that values individual achievement, autonomy, and charm, the package that narcissists present can seem rather attractive and the bearers of this package quite pleased with themselves. What is more, people who are genuinely competent and talented and smart enough to present themselves effectively may actually succeed in making their way in the world. This would parallel the finding that while most quick decision-makers get themselves into trouble because their failures earn them the label of "impulsive," individuals who combine fast response with effective response may not be seen as "impulsive" at all, but rather as "brilliant" [21].

Of course, Sedikides and his colleagues are not the only and last word on the benefits and costs of narcissism. For one thing, their research involves young people (college students mainly) – and they will grow out of this, as we all learn, often to our shock and amazement. My mentor, Urie Bronfenbrenner began his critique of mainstream psychology in the early 1970s as "the study of college sophomores in unfamiliar situations" [22]. A more systematic version of which was published by David Sears in 1986 under the title, "College Sophomores in the Laboratory:

Influences of a Narrow Data Base on Social Psychology's View of Human Nature," [23] and concluded that "compared with adults, college students are likely to have less-crystallized attitudes, less-formulated senses of self, stronger cognitive skills, stronger tendencies to comply with authority, and more unstable peer relationships. The laboratory situation is likely to exaggerate all these differences" (p. 515).

This might be quite relevant here because the limitations of narcissism as a basis for living a satisfying and successful life may not emerge for most people until they are past youth and young adulthood, into middle age. That's an important caveat, captured well, I think, by *A New Yorker* cartoon some years ago that has a man wistfully saying to his friend, "I just realized I am now too old to be 'the youngest anything' anymore." To some degree then, narcissism in a person's life may go the way of many of youth's irritating habits: if time heals all wounds, it also wounds all heels (and gives them a chance to become a better person for that).

Where does narcissism come from? As with most human behavior, the core answer is "it depends." It depends upon the accumulation of biological, psychological, social, and cultural influences. Like most human traits, narcissism seems to have its roots in biology, family, and culture. Studies have shown that there is a genetic component to narcissism: identical twins are more likely to share this trait than are nonidentical twins and other siblings [24]. But a simple reading of this as biological determinism would be as wrong here as it is elsewhere.

Like the biological foundations for intelligence, the actual contribution of genetic influences to the development of narcissism depends upon whether the psychosocial environment passively allows biological predisposition to flower into adult personality, or systematically works to blunt those biological predispositions – or whether it nurtures and encourages them. Context matters. For example, a 1970 analysis of data available to that point indicated that the correlation in IQ scores of identical twins raised in similar communities was 0.89, but the correlation of IQ scores for identical twins raised in *dissimilar* communities was only 0.29 [22]! Does genetic predisposition predict IQ development? It depends. Does biology predict narcissism? It too depends.

What about family? The standard explanation regarding family origins not surprisingly focuses on two things. The first is a parent who dotes on the child and thus engenders a sense of entitlement and a habit of self-promotion. The second is a pattern of emotional coldness. As psychologists Jeffrey Young and Catherine Flanagan conclude in their contribution to *Disorders of Narcissism*: "One typical origin for narcissism involves a child who is overvalued by the mother, is undervalued by the father and experiences minimal unselfish love from either or both." (pp. 246–247) [24]. The overvaluation builds up the child's agency, while the lack of unselfish love interferes with communion. Both speak to the critical role played by genuine acceptance in creating positive human development.

As I noted in Chap. 2, anthropologist Ronald Rohner and his colleagues [25] have studied parental acceptance and rejection in cultures around the world. They find that across cultures and societies, children thrive when accepted, and wither and distort when rejected, so much so that Rohner calls rejection a "psychological malignancy." On average, parental rejection (vs. acceptance) accounts for about

25% of the difference in whether or not children develop antisocial or otherwise troubled development. This makes it one of the most powerful effects observed in human psychology and, of course, does the same for acceptance, making it too "one of the most powerful effects observed in human psychology."

What about the school? The educational process and the institutions that house it play a role in narcissism, to be sure. How? When the school promotes glorification of self over being embedded in the group, it runs the risk of stimulating and feeding narcissism. Similarly, when schools glorify individual victory over group coopera-tion, they run the risk of stimulating aggrandizement and self-inflation [26].

What about culture as a whole? Culture matters a great deal. The seeds of narcis-sism that may come from biological predispositions are watered in family socializa-tion, but then, culture can play an important role in whether those seeds blossom or wither. This blossoming happens when the messages coming to children, youth, and adults focus on self-validation for its own sake, on glorification of self-indulgence in the life of "exemplars." It comes when the cult of celebrity prevails, in which "being rich and famous" is the stated goal of many people and the subject of blatant validation in the mass media, and in the boosting of individuality – even at the expense of social connection [27].

Seligman has something to say about this. "Get in touch with your feelings," shout the self-esteem peddlers in our society. Our youth have absorbed this message, and believing it has produced a generation of narcissists whose major concern, not surprisingly, "is with how they feel." (p. 118). [4] A younger reader might think this sounds a bit curmudgeonly – just the kind of thing that a 60-something-year-old man might say about "kids today." Seligman is 5 years older than I am, so he was the same age as I am now when he wrote this, thus I realize I am open to the same charges when I say I tend to agree with him on this point.

But there is some research to back up Seligman's curmudgeonly critique of kids today, according to Jean Twenge and Keith Campbell in their book *The Narcissism Epidemic: Living in the Age of Entitlement* [28]. They cite surveys indicating that narcissism *has* been on the rise – particularly among young people, and especially among young women – since the 1980s. At present, they say, one in four college students is reporting a score of 20 or more on the Narcissistic Personality Inventory used by Sedikitis and his colleagues [20] (although his group found an average score of only 14), and one in ten young adults (and 1 in 16 people overall) meets the criteria for the clinical diagnosis of Narcissistic Personality Disorder.

But culture can play an opposite role, as evident in the life story of the 14th Dalai Lama. Chosen as a young child to become the spiritual and political leader of Tibet because he was thought to be the reincarnation of the 13th Dalai Lama, 2-year-old Lhamo Dhondup would appear to have been at high risk for becoming a raging narcissist as he was transformed into Tenzin Gyatso, the Dalai Lama. Singled out as transcendently special by the Buddhist clergy, this little boy began a series of experiences that could turn anyone's head. He was moved from the rough and tumble world of his home to the opulence of the Potala Palace in Lhasa where he was venerated as a spiritual being. He received virtually unlimited adult attention – even adoration.

But Tenzin Gyatzo did not become a narcissist. He was immersed in a culture that protected him from this fate by training him for a life of service and humility, by teaching him Buddhist principles and concepts about the nature of "self" and the folly of "attachment" that protected him, and by involving him in a daily practice of meditation that gave him a core of Bakan's communion and a profound wisdom about the follies of self-absorption. We should all be so fortunate. I wish I were.

Like many adults, I carry with me every day the challenges of healing my wounded inner child, of coming home to my earliest self and reclaiming my right to feel safe, cared for, and worthwhile, and doing so in a way that does not elicit the opposite problem of what might be called reactive or defensive narcissism (i.e., having an exaggerated concept of self-worth and self-esteem to compensate for an underlying feeling of unworthiness). Reading Jeffrey Young and Catherine Flanagan's [24] analysis of the family conditions that spawn narcissism, I felt like I was hearing a description of my own family. Reading Wendy Behary's account of loneliness and shame in the psyche of narcissists, I felt like I was reading my autobiography. Reading about temperamental risk factors for narcissism, I feel like I am looking in the mirror. Considering the cultural foundations for narcissism, I see them around me – and know I have often swallowed and embodied them.

I must admit to being drawn to my narcissist within, although I think my issues with Asperger's, coupled with my high achievement motivation, are really the culprit. I do think that I have been on the road to recovery for some time and, I think, I have always been a relatively nice narcissist, a socially conscious narcissist, and usually a kind and generous narcissist. "Hi, I'm Jim, and it's been X days since I thought of myself in grandiose terms at the expense of others." My score on the Narcissistic Personality Inventory is lower now [15] than it would have been only a few short years ago (projecting backward I can easily imagine scoring 30).

When I took the NPA Personality Test developed by psychiatrist A. M. Benis (a lengthier and more complex instrument than the NPI, which seeks to identify several possible personality types) [29], the results showed that the probability of me having a narcissistic personality was 1.0 (as opposed to a small fraction of that for all the mixed patterns and for the other two types in the Benis system). On the graph, my Narcissism score (in red on the printout) reached to the top of the scale. Aren't I special?

In my 60s now, I feel the press of time to do something about my narcissism. One tactic has been to work on building up my commitment to group participation and commitment to others ("communion" in Bakan's conception). This is easier said than done, of course, and can only take things so far. For example, when I volunteered to help serve dinner on Christmas Day at the Salvation Army, it was a struggle not to take charge, to be charming with the other volunteers and the diners, and to make this service a story about me. The fact that I am engaged in the struggle is the good news; the fact that it is so hard is the ongoing problem.

Every child grows up with unfinished business from childhood. For some of us, it is coming to terms with an imperious father; for others it centers on our issues of abandonment. Whatever it is, children do what they must to create a tentative working solution that allows them to get on with the process of becoming an adult in the world.

For me, the unfinished business of childhood is learning to work with my Asperger's traits to open my heart to the world, experience the present without always looking to the future, feel things more directly. As a "recovering narcissist," my goal is to allow ambition to take a back seat, for compassion to be more than an intellectual exercise, and for the primacy of relationships to flow through my life.

My mother taught me a great deal about how to be competent and successful in the world. She is a smart and competitive woman who was frustrated by the ways in which the limitations of her history (growing up in the 1930s), class (working), culture (in England), and temperament (shy about public performance) had prevented her from living a "big" life (a life she found only in old age when she became a celebrity senior citizen in her home town – winning awards, accolades, and praise for her triumphs). She taught me to be ambitious, as much for her own sake as my own, and with it came all the paraphernalia of narcissism – a sense of entitlement, a strong competitive drive, high self-esteem, and a tactical approach to life. Of course, this was precisely the kind of "social skills training" that allowed me to escape many of the lifelong limitations that often come along with Asperger's.

My appreciation for the role of ambition in driving my life has been slow in coming (self-reflection was not a virtue but a curse in my mother's book, of course, nor is it a trait that Asperger's promotes). It wasn't until middle age that I began to have an inkling of what taking up the mantle of ambition in the context of being so emotionally inept had cost me. One pivotal moment came when talking with my daughter Joanna when she was in her early twenties, when I found myself cataloging her many "advantages" as a child of well-educated and affluent parents (when compared to my own financial and status struggles as a blue-collar child).

Unlike me, she had never had an unemployed father. Unlike me, she had highly educated parents who could show her the ropes that led to her Ivy League college education. Unlike me, she had traveled abroad and been exposed to "high culture" from an early age. I was taken aback when she rebuked me by saying, "Yes dad, but you had something I didn't have, ambition." I credit my mother with instilling in me that ambition. But it came at a cost. Doesn't everything?

I started life as a sensitive child, not in the sense that I was naturally empathic, but in the sense that I was easily overwhelmed: I cried rivers each September when elementary school started and when I was sent away to a 2-day-long summer camp. I was highly sensitive about my speech impediment – a lisp. I was so shy about speaking in public that I was immobilized when stood up in front of a group. But I "triumphed" over my sensitivity by social skills training and a lot of "force of will."

I set my feelings aside (such as they were) as a way to overcome challenges and went on to fulfill my mother's ambitions for me. Looking back on it, I think the only way I could take on the mantle of her unfulfilled ambition was to shut down the overwhelmed child and exile him to some silent place in my secret self. This is why the first time I heard John Bradshaw talk about "reclaiming and healing the wounded inner child" [30], I wept in recognition of what I had lost so long ago. Fifty years later I am coming back to that little boy I left behind, and walking with Hope and Dharma plays a big role in that process.

Looking at all that now, I think this "inner child betrayed" explains a great deal about the way I developed, in light of the temperamental issues I brought to the situation as a child dealing with Asperger's issues. It illuminates many of the worst things in my life – the common theme of which is a kind of coldheartedness that I see in my first marriage, in the shallowness of my adult friendships, in the strains in my relationships with Josh and Joanna in the years following the divorce that ended their "normal" family and with my stepson Eric in the years following my marriage to his mother, and in the challenges I have faced in my second marriage, in short in my own form of narcissism. Until recently self-help books and therapists have not been all that helpful – an illustration, I think, of the old adage that "you can lead a horse to water, but you can't make him drink." Dogs? They are more likely to drink. Walking with Hope and Dharma has helped me recognize and deal with all this.

Many observers of human–dog relationships have noted that one of the attractive features of dogs (from a human's point of view) is that a dog is open to molding, bonding, and simply being together without the kind of evaluation that humans face so often at school, in peer groups, at work, and in our families. This may even extend to healing the "inner child" in adults, for decades of research demonstrates that this process of unconditional acceptance is undeniably crucial for healthy human development.

Seligman [4] focuses on the dangers of the touchy-feely, easy-pleasure principle of the younger generation, and Twenge and Campbell [28] focus on the risky core belief that self-admiration will improve your life. In addition, there is the narcissistic nature of American history itself, based upon what historians have called "exceptionalism." [31]. When historians refer our "historical exceptionalism," they mean that we tend to view our history as unique and special, and to reject the idea that we are like everyone else, as a people and as a country. It is a rare politician who can refrain from saying "This is the greatest nation on Earth."

Many would go so far as to say this is the greatest nation that has ever existed, unique among all countries. In the nineteenth century we proclaimed our divinely inspired "manifest destiny" to expand across the North American continent – and in some people's minds across the world. America rests on the belief that we are above and beyond the rest of the world – "We're Number One!" – and therefore entitled to exceptional status. Sound familiar? Substitute "I" for "the United States" and you get the message: the theme of exceptionalism reverberates down through the decades of American history, providing a constant infusion of cultural support for narcissism in the psyche of individual people who are inclined to believe "I'm Number One!"

And there is more. In another of their studies, Sedikides and his colleagues [32] offered a provocative analysis of one of the downsides of narcissism, namely, the way marketers can manipulate potential consumers by playing to their grandiosity. They called their report "The I that buys: narcissists as consumers," and describe it thus: "Which people are most swayed by self-image motives and hence most likely to make consumer choices in line with those motives? We contend that the answer is narcissists, individuals who see themselves, and who want others to see them, as special, superior, and entitled, and who are prone to exhibitionism and vanity. We hypothesize that narcissists will, to validate their excessively positive self-views, strive to purchase the high-prestige products (i.e., expensive, exclusive, new, and flashy). In so doing, they will regulate their own esteem by increasing their apparent status and consequently earning others' admiration and envy. We also hypothesize that narcissists will show greater interest in the symbolic than utilitarian value of products, and will exhibit, even controlling for self-esteem, more pronounced self-enhancement phenomena, such as endowment and self-signaling effects" [32].

It's a bit deliciously ironic to think of narcissists being manipulated (I guess I should say *other* narcissists). In my case, an ideological commitment to living a materially simple life tends to protect me. Given their (our) penchant for manipulating others, there is a certain justice to the results of this study, but it also speaks of the fact that there is much in our culture and our society that feeds narcissism. The constant message, "you are what you buy" is strong and corrupting, and perhaps narcissists are simply more vulnerable to it than other people (said at the risk of feeding the sense of "specialness" characteristic of narcissism in the first place).

In this sense, narcissism is "rational" for the individual – and this is why Sedikides and his colleagues found it to be associated with good mental health (and even good marriages in some situations). But ultimately it is destructive for the community, in this case the other people who share the world with the narcissist (whether the narcissist acknowledges that or not). Sedikides and his colleagues use a powerful metaphor to communicate this: "The mind of a narcissist is like a sports utility vehicle. It is great to be in the driving seat, but fellow motorists must watch out, lest a collision with this mobile fortress demolish their more humble hatchbacks" (p. 412) [32]. In this sense, it is as rational to be a narcissist as it is to drive an SUV.

Reading this I think of two things. The first is what ecologist Garrett Hardin called "The Tragedy of the Commons" [33] in a famous article published in the journal *Science* in 1968. Hardin showed how the net effect of individuals acting independently in their own self-interest can lead to collective destruction. The "commons" here is a metaphor that refers to the fact that in a situation where grazing lands are held in common by a community, there must be strong collective rules to restrain self-interest. Without these rules, it is in the rational self-interest of each person to graze as many cows as possible on the communal land because for that individual, it is "free." But the collective effect of each individual acting on the basis of this reasonable calculation is overgrazing that results in the destruction of the commons, and eventually disaster for each of the "rational" individuals who caused the problem in the first place, Sounds like Wall Street.

The second thing is the debates about carbon emissions and global warming issues, and Keith Campbell and his colleagues [34] have conducted a small study to demonstrate that narcissists are particularly vulnerable to the behavior that leads to the tragedy of the commons. In their study, students were asked to play the role of a forestry company CEO – in competition with three others harvesting from the same forest. Those scoring high on the Narcissism Scale "won" in the short run (by cutting down more trees). But the more Narcissists who played the game, the quicker the entire forest disappeared and all lost out: maximizing profit while still preserving resources requires more cooperative, less narcissistic individuals. More people won in the long run when "the participants were less entitled." (p. 240) [34].

As each narcissist serves his or her individual agenda, the world as a whole grows sadder. You can hear this in the laments of the many Web sites and books devoted to "living with a narcissist" in one form or another. Narcissism is unhelpful in many of the most important social contexts in human experience, such as maintaining long-term relationships and taking empathic and compassionate care of other living beings. So conclude psychologists Keith Campbell and Joshua Foster based upon their review of the evidence [35].

This is why more than 40 years ago, David Bakan insisted that "The mitigation of agency with communion, therefore, provides a proper goal of the individual throughout life." [13]. For the good of the human condition – indeed the condition of all sentient beings on the planet – the forces of ego and self must make peace with the forces of compassion, empathy, and connection. Narcissists take heed. I am listening.

There are attempts to help narcissists get over themselves and on the road to recover, however. A Web-based community called http://www.experienceproject.com hosts a site called "I am a narcissist" and bills it as "read true personal stories, chat and get advice from a group of 60 people who all say 'I am a Narcissist.'" The site's page gives you a choice to push one of three buttons: "Me too," "Not Me," or "Plan To." Selfhelpmagazine.com offers advice on how to proceed with actually establishing a Narcissists Anonymous group. I think that it would be hard to sustain a Narcissists Anonymous Group – hard-core narcissists could not or would not tolerate being anonymous, but if they could, they would already be starting on the road to recovery as I hope I am, with the help of Wendy Behary's book Disarming the Narcissist [18].

The famous philosophical comic strip character Pogo is most famous for the line, "We have met the enemy and he is us." For a recovering narcissist, perhaps the better rendering is "We have met the enemy and he is I (…and isn't he special)." The fundamental problem is a *self* problem and that poses some real challenges for a positive psychology, as Buddhist psychoanalyst Polly Young-Eisendrath recognizes in her book *The Self Esteem Trap: Raising Confident and Compassionate Kids in an Age of Self-importance* [27].

Seligman's positive psychology has a lot to say about self related issues. The index includes "self-absorption," "self-congratulation," "self-control," "self-esteem," "self-esteem movement," "self help movement," and "self-overvaluation," but no "self" [4]. That may be a problem, since perhaps the only ultimate solution to narcissism – for individual narcissists and for the narcissistic society as a whole – is to be found in the very concept of self.

What is the antidote to narcissism? From Seligman's perspective – one that I share in large part – the task is to recognize the path from ego-driven self to a more communion-driven self and a self that focuses on "gratifications" rather than "pleasures." In Seligman's terms, "It is the total absorption, the suspension of consciousness, and the flow that the gratifications produce that defines liking these activities – not the presence of pleasure. Total immersion, in fact, blocks consciousness, and emotions are complete absent. This distinction is the difference between the good life and the pleasant life." (p. 111) [4].

Doing good things – temporarily "losing yourself" – is a step in the right direction, of course, particularly if it stimulates and enhances communion. What Zen Buddhist Thich Nhat Hanh [36] and others, like the psychologist Ellen Langer, call "mindfulness" is another [37]. For Langer, the goal is to reduce mindlessness and promote mindfulness. For Thich Nhat Hanh, the focus is on being fully present all the time. Actually, even the phrase "all the time" is an error when discussing mindfulness in Buddhist terms, since living in the past and the future rather than in the present moment is part of the problem – no, as Thich Nhat Hanh would say, it *is* the problem. These approaches can take us a long way (me included). But where do we go (where do I go) to find a solution to the underlying problem of self upon which narcissism is built?

One of the "jokes" on the Lisa Scott Web site mentioned earlier offers one clue: "What do you call a narcissist who can graciously accept criticism or blame? Dead." In one sense that is a rather grim prognosis. In another, it may be a very positive clue, since it is the answer to the question "death of what" that provides the positive answer.

I was looking again at the index for Seligman's book "Authentic Happiness," and found Dawson, S. 281, Deci, E. 294, decision latitude, 179–180, 181–182. Something is missing: death (dying is not there either, between Dwyer, C. 278 and dysphorias, *see* negative emotions). [4] In one sense this is quite understandable. After all, what place does death have in a positive psychology? What place indeed?

The German existentialist philosopher Martin Heidegger, who wrote one of the most important books of philosophy of the twentieth century, *Being and Time*, [38] insisted that until one had contemplated "non-being," one was not prepared to understand being. Of course Heidegger's bona fides as a spokesperson for understanding human development are compromised by the fact that he joined the Nazi Party in 1933 and embraced Adolf Hitler. Nonetheless, I think that he was on the mark in understanding that life without death didn't make full sense for understanding the human condition. At least, I think this is what he was saying.

Some 40+ years ago I spent long hours in the library when I was an undergraduate trying to read, let alone understand, the 592-page *Being and Time*. I often looked to the footnotes for clarification, only to find they were in Greek and/or Latin. It would be 30 years until William Blattner wrote his book *Heidegger's Being and Time: A Reader's Guide* [39]. I do recall actually believing that I understood two consecutive paragraphs, one day in 1967, and made a note of it in the margin of my book: "I think I understand this!!!!"

Heidegger is not alone in this insistence that embracing death is a prerequisite for embracing life fully. It is a tenet of Christianity and Buddhism as well as a core principle of existentialism generally. Some of this is purely cognitive in the sense that it is difficult if not impossible to understand something fully unless you are aware of and understand it's opposite. This belief is captured in the old saw, "how would a fish describe water?" Since fish do not know air, they cannot appreciate fully the characteristics of water (assuming a fish could describe anything, what with their very tiny brains and very, very short-term memories).

I trust the Dalai Lama on most matters, so when he says that one of the benefits of his monkish existence is that he can spend a few hours early each morning contemplating nonbeing, I believe he must be on to something. Why? Because contemplating and encountering death is an eye-opening experience (or at least it can be). Not everyone who contemplates death comes away with an enhanced and renewed zest for a meaningful life, of course, but those who have studied this matter most intensely, namely, the practitioners of meditation and deep prayer, attest to its productive power. This is at the core of Buddhism.

That this is difficult is no surprise to anyone who has attempted it. In fact, the human brain appears to have evolved to specialize in looking to the future. According to psychologist Daniel Gilbert's delightful book *Stumbling on Happiness*, [40] the emergence of the frontal lobe of our brains is the defining difference between human beings and other beings on the planet, and that the principal function of the frontal lobe is future-oriented mental activities. He writes of the challenge we face and why it takes such profound effort to accomplish mindfulness, "Not to think about the future requires that we convince our frontal lobe not to do what it was designed to do, and like a heart that is told not to beat, it naturally resists this suggestion." (p. 17) Research reveals that about 12% of our daily thoughts are about the future – more than we think about the past or the present. This sets the terms for meditation and other efforts to dislodge us from the future.

Remember that Buddhism is not only a religion, but is also – some would say primarily – a psychology, a very positive psychology. It is in large part a psychology of self as well as a positive psychology of happiness. It may seem ironic, then, that for this positive psychology of self, a core concept is anatta or "no self." Indeed, the "death" of self is one of the principal avenues to happiness. This arises from the Four Noble Truths mentioned in an earlier chapter: the root of suffering is attachment, and attachment to self is the biggest problem of all.

Two psychotherapists who have grasped this are Jett Psaris and Marlena Lyons [41]. In their book "Undefended Love" they put it this way: "In the healthy process of maturing, we would move from compulsion about determining and controlling how we get our needs met to increasing levels of acceptance of what life offers us as sufficient. As enlightened masters demonstrate, at the most evolved level we do not need things to be other than they are – we have no preferences. Everything carries equal value. This continuum also reflects what happens as we move from close relationship to the deep fulfillment of an undefended and unrehearsed partnership" (p. 141).

Simply confronting death doesn't guarantee the wisdom to give up the self-centered arrogance and insensitivity that poison human relationships for narcissists. My former father-in-law's life is a testament to that. He spent the last year of World War II in a German prisoner of war camp, after having been captured when his plane (a B-24 bomber) was shot down on his first mission over Germany in 1944. He kept a diary – written with a pencil on cigarette papers – about the privation he experienced and the fear of death that haunted him and his fellow prisoners. Because of this experience, he resolved that he would never be hungry again, and as a desperate celebration of surviving had bacon and eggs for breakfast every day for the rest of his life – until he died of lung cancer in his early 60s, a condition that was worsened by his heart disease and heavy drinking – another fatal celebration of living, if not life.

But more to the point here, he was a classic narcissist who met all the diagnostic criteria for narcissistic personality disorder. Indeed, all those "jokes" about narcissism I reported earlier could have been written specifically about him. He was shockingly egocentric, domineering, arrogant, insensitive to the needs of others, and at the same time superficially charming and competent. I knew him for almost 20 years, and I saw and heard how he made the lives of his spouse and children emotional Hell, all the while using his superficial charm to create a successful life as a salesman for an engineering firm.

He never had a dog, and that means he never experienced the death of a beloved canine companion. Perhaps if he had he would lived a wiser life, making better use of his encounter with death in World War II to shake him loose from his preoccupation with the grandiosity of himself. Perhaps loving a dog, a dog that would die before he did could have changed him, perhaps given him another chance to use his World War II encounter with death to stimulate wisdom rather than mindless hedonism in the service of self. Perhaps it could have stimulated the spiritual awakening that he needed but never achieved in this lifetime. Perhaps not. But it worth contemplating this educative role that dying dogs can perform, in addition to the many other exemplary services they perform for their human companions.

There is a natural course to the relationships between humans and dogs – to have and to hold, to love and to cherish, through sickness and health, till death do us part. When the natural course of this relationship happens, there is a peacefulness to its ending in a dog's death that can contribute to the human's sense of trust and confidence in the circle of life, and move us off center, away from our precious selves. Of course, like many human-to-human marriages, the relationships of humans and dogs do not always follow this ideal path.

Some dogs die too young, unexpectedly and traumatically. It is estimated that tens of thousands of dogs are hit by cars each year. Dogs get lost or are given away. It is estimated that some seven million dogs enter animal shelters each year [43]. Many of these are lost, and less than 15% of these are returned to their owners. Thus, many thousands of people – children included – lose their dogs each year – because they run away, because they are given away, because they are stolen, or because of family disruption that separates people from their dogs. Preventing these losses and helping children deal with them when they occur is an important issue, and an issue that can reverberate for a lifetime. Thirty-two-year-old Bob's story speaks volumes.

"I was 12 when our dog Corrie disappeared. We were driving cross country for our vacation and we stopped at a rest stop on the highway in Ohio. Before anyone realized it was happening Corrie bolted across the parking lot and into the woods. I don't know what he saw or what he smelled, but he was gone. We called for him for more than two hours and then my dad said we had to go. We put up a notice at the rest stop and even called the local SPCA, but we never heard from anyone. It's been 20 years, and I have had other dogs since then, but there it still hurts to remember how we lost Corrie."

Because the maximum typical life span of a dog is only about 14 years, most people who enter into companion relationships with dogs will eventually have to deal with the death of that dog. Nearly four million dogs living in American families die each year [42]. When and how this death occurs can matter a great deal.

But the death of a dog can teach a child important lessons about dying – and about life. My daughter Joanna's 14-year relationship with our dog Abby is just such a story.

"When we got Abby, she was so small that she fit into a beer box. She was the runt of the litter and my mom thought she would die. Abby decided to live the day she met ice cream in the back seat of the car. We always got her own 'baby size' cone after that. Abby was always there from the time I was 7 until I was 21, and she became playmate, horse substitute, and role model. Her biggest vice, like many people, was sweets (as we should have figured out by her will to live coming from soft serve ice cream). Once she ate an entire plate of brownies off the coffee table! One year she jumped up on the kitchen counter and ate half my dad's Father's Day cake (we iced over that part and ate it anyway). If you weren't watching, she'd take edible things out of the hands of small children, but always politely and gently. We spent our summers on an island in a lake in the woods of northern New York State, so for 2 months each year it was just me, my older brother, my mom and dad, and Abby, so she was my main friend. A couple of summers we won the 'best costume' contest at the local County Fair; one year we both dressed up as cowboys. I taught her to jump jumps, just like a horse. Looking back on it, it probably wasn't the best thing for her weak back legs, but she never complained. I would spend hours throwing balls or sticks into the water for her to retrieve – both she and I enjoying every time she splashed down into the water off the dock. When she died, I realized what a constant she'd been in my life and how you never really appreciate what you have until it's gone. Other dogs will come and go, but they will always be compared to, and fall short of, the standard set by Abby. She was a saint and the best dog that will ever be."

The poignancy of dying dogs is a recurrent theme in human accounts of their canine friends. The biological realities of life span force that issue, of course, but the psychological and spiritual ramifications of losing a canine companion in this manner reflect the intensity of the bonds. Two men who have captured this intensity are John Grogan [43] – author of *Marley and Me* – and Ted Kerasote [44] – author of *Merle's Door*. Having read a lot of dog memoirs, I would say that these two are the best, and I think that it is not coincidental that both authors are men: dogs give us men license to be more fully human by legitimizing our emotional lives as few other beings can and do.

Men are trained to be closed-mouthed about their feelings (and perhaps even to lose some of their innate capacity to feel these emotions at all). Hardly a relationship book goes by without some commentary or interview transcript testimony to this protective closeness in men (and to some degree boys). Seligman recognizes this [4], noting research that demonstrates women experience both more negative and more positive emotions than men do. In their books about the boy code, psychologists Michael Thompson and Dan Kindlon (*Raising Cain*) [45] and William Pollock (*Real Boys*) [46] comment on how boys learn to close down their emotional expressiveness for fear of seeming unmanly.

A recent compendium of writings on "the feminine ethic of care" [47] documents this line: sexism and speciesism do tend to go together – and always have. As one historian of animal care puts it in speaking of Descartes' era – the seventeenth century – "Although there were notable campaigners for compassion towards animals, the overall effect of this anthropocentric world view was that cruelty to animals was relatively commonplace." (p. 180) [47]. It was a man's world, and the worst of masculinity dominated the world of dogs – and other animals (and women, and children). But this is not the whole story, however.

In today's world, there are some very limited and ritualized settings or contexts where male emotional expressiveness is culturally permitted. One is sports, where demonstrations of emotion – hugging and crying, for example – are sanctioned. The other is in relationship with animals – mostly dogs. This opens men to the world women more naturally inhabit, through custom and temperament, the real world of human emotion.

In fact, their relationships with dogs are one of the few that permit males to develop and express their softer, more nurturing and expressive side. Reporting on her observation of how a very manly man and his young son cared for their sick dog in the waiting room of a vet's office, psychologist Gail Melson [48] writes, "I had been watching a 10-year-old boy, one, moreover, who looked like a poster child for all-American masculinity. Both he and his John Wayne-lookalike father had been in tender public embrace of a small, needy creature. Where else were boys or men to be seen displaying such gentle care giving? The answer seemed obvious – nowhere." (p. 2) Perhaps it is significant that the death of a dog is such a powerful heart opener for men like Merle's Kerasote and Marley's Grogan.I feel this myself. It is in relationship with our dogs Hope and Dharma that I feel most free emotionally. Just contemplating their deaths opens the floodgates of emotion that are so often locked for me, and in so doing open me more to the costs of self that are inherent in my narcissism. Like my daughter Joanna, I remember the death of Abby as a time of immense emotional release that had profound psychological reverberations, drawing a measure of positivity from a situation that was locked into negativity.

By the time Abby died, Joanna's mother and I were divorced – and on anything but good terms. Our infrequent face-to-face encounters ranged from stiff and forced to hostile and cold. Abby lived with Joanna's mother at that point and just visited with me occasionally, and when the vet advised that the 14-year-old dog was failing fast, it was decided to end her painful last days as humanely as possible, and at home.

To her credit, Joanna's mother invited me to be there for the last moments. I was grateful for that opportunity. I held and stroked Abby as the vet administered the lethal injection that literally put her to final sleep. When it was over, I laid her silent still head down, got up, and then spontaneously kissed my ex-wife on the cheek as I left – the first positive contact we had in the years since the divorce. Love of dogs can do that. But it can't do everything.

The shock of confronting death can be a good start for finding a positive path, one not consumed by narcissism. Confronting death is no guarantee of enlightenment – or even that one will be on the path to enlightenment. But confronting death can be a form of what might be called psychological chemotherapy, in the sense that it uses the poison of trauma to defeat a greater threat to well-being posed by narcissistic attachment to self. Like chemotherapy, however, trauma can have serious side effects, as we saw earlier.

Is there a way to get the benefits of confronting death without the noxious side effects of traumatic chemotherapy? I think that we can see that in the meditative disciplines that take a more systematic and gentle approach to the Anatta (not self or no self). As one Buddhist teacher of American origin – Thanissaro Bhikkhu [49] – put it:

"Stress should be comprehended, its cause abandoned, its cessation realized, and the path to its cessation developed. These duties form the context in which the Anatta doctrine is best understood. If you develop the path of virtue, concentration, and discernment to a state of calm well-being and use that calm state to look at experience in terms of the Noble Truths, the questions that occur to the mind are not "Is there a self? What is myself?" but rather "Am I suffering stress because I'm holding onto this particular phenomenon? Is it really me, myself, or mine? If it's stressful but not really me or mine, why hold on?" These last questions merit straightforward answers, as they then help you to comprehend stress and to chip away at the attachment and clinging – the residual sense of self-identification – that cause it, until ultimately all traces of self-identification are gone and all that's left is limitless freedom. In this sense, the Anatta teaching is not a doctrine of no-self, but a not-self strategy for shedding suffering by letting go of its cause, leading to the highest, undying happiness. At that point, questions of self, no-self, and not-self fall aside. Once there's the experience of such total freedom, where would there be any concern about what's experiencing it, or whether or not it's a self?"

Avoiding dualities is the goal here, as it is in the spiritual practice developed by the Christian St. Ignatius of Loyola. In Ignatian spirituality the goal is to attain an open acceptance predicated on divine trust. It is a trust that foregoes attachment to the ups and downs of daily life – neither consolation nor desolation, but rather detachment from worldly outcome. It speaks for a commitment to social justice (communion) and a self embedded in the positive gratifications of good living devoid of attachments to material illusions.

And here, I think, is where Buddhism, positive psychology, and the kind of Christian spirituality represented by St. Ignatius of Loyola meet, in aligning with the positive forces in the universe – the big universe of "the world" and the little universe within. They align in giving yourself up to communion, to flow, to action on behalf of the good, rather than focusing on momentary pleasures or constructions of ego. At their best, Buddhism, positive psychology, and Ignatian Christian spirituality are all *practices* rather than ideologies or systems of belief. All three imply a state of grace that one earns through efforts to construct a pattern of gratifying constructive and playful activities – in the case of positive psychology – meditative practice that puts the temptations of misguided attachments into perspective – in the case of Buddhism and Ignatian spirituality. As a recovering narcissist myself, I feel strongly the need to bring to bear this practice on existence, on my existence. As a member of a narcissistic society, I think that they offer us collective redemption, a positive path to meaningfulness – with a large dose of happiness thrown in for good measure.

References

1. Bowlby, J. (1969) Attachment, Vol. 1 of Attachment and loss. London: Hogarth Press. New York: Basic Books; Harmondsworth: Penguin (1971).
2. http://www.mayoclinic.com/health/reactive-attachment-disorder/ds00988.
3. Santrock, J. (2008) Life-span development. New York, NY: McGraw-Hill.
4. Seligman, M. (2004) Authentic happiness. New York, NY: Free Press.
5. http://www.selfpsychology.org/whatis.htm.
6. Webb, W. (1952) The great frontier. Austin, TX: The University of Texas.
7. Riesman, D. Glazer, N. and Denney, R. (1950) The lonely crowd. New Haven, CT: Yale University Press.
8. Slater, P. (1970) The pursuit of loneliness. Boston, MA: Beacon Press.
9. Putnam, R. (2000) Bowling alone. New York, NY: Putnam.
10. Caccioppo, J. and Patrick, W. (2008) Loneliness: human nature and the need for connection. New York, NY: Putnam.
11. Rotenberg, M. (1977) Alienating individualism and reciprocal individualism: a cross-cultural conceptualization. Humanistic Psychology. 17. 3–17.
12. Garbarino, J. (1977) The price of privacy. Child Welfare. 56. 565–575.
13. Bakan, D. (1966) The duality of human existence. Boston, MA: Beacon Press.
14. Buss, D. (1980) Unmitigated agency and unmitigated communion: an analysis of negative components of masculinity and femininity. Sex Roles. 22. 555–568.
15. American Psychiatric Association (2000) DSM-IV. Washington, DC: American Psychiatric Association.
16. MacFarquhar, L. (2009) The kindest cut? The New Yorker. July 27, 2009, p. 39ff.
17. http://www.kidney.org/.
18. Behary, W. (2008) Disarming the narcissist. Oakland, CA: New Harbinger Publications.
19. Martinez-Lewis, L. (2008) Freeing yourself from the narcissist in your life. New York, NY: Tarcher.
20. Sedikides, C., Rudich, E. A. Gregg, A. P. Kumashiro, M. and Rusbult, C. (2004) Are normal narcissists psychologically healthy? Self-esteem matters. Journal of Personality and Social Psychology. 87. 400–416.
21. Sheppard, L. and Vernon, P. (2008) Intelligence and speed of information-processing: a review of 50 years of research. Personality and Individual Differences. 44. 535–551.
22. Bronfenbrenner, U. (1979) The ecology of human development. Cambridge, MA: Harvard University Press.
23. Sears, D. (1986) College sophomores in the laboratory; influences of a narrow data base on social psychology's view of human nature. Journal of Personal and Social Psychology. 51. 515–530.
24. Young, J. and Flanagan, C. (2000) Schema-focused therapy for narcissistic patients. In E. Ronningstam (Ed.) Disorders of Narcissism. Washington, DC: American Psychiatric Press. pp. 239–265.
25. Rohner, R. (1975) They love me, they love me not. Princeton, NJ: Human Area Files Press.
26. Garbarino, J. (1994) Raising children in a socially toxic environment. San Francisco, CA: Jossey-Bass.
27. Young-Eisendrath, P. (2009) The self esteem trap: raising confident and compassionate kids in an age of self-importance. Boston, MA: Little, Brown.
28. Twenge, J. and Campbell, K. (2010) The narcissism epidemic: living in an age of entitlement. New York, NY: Free Press.
29. Benis, A.M. http://personalitytest.homestead.com/.
30. Bradshaw, J. (1992) Homecoming: reclaiming and healing your inner child. New York, NY: Bantam.
31. Ross, D. (1991) The origins of American social science. New York, NY: Cambridge University Press.

32. Sedikides, C. Gregg, A. Cisek, and Hart, C. (2007) The I that buys: narcissists as consumers. Journal of Consumer Psychology. 17. 254–257.
33. Hardin, G. (1968) Tragedy of the commons. Science. 162. 1243–1248.
34. Campbell, K., Bush, C. Brunell, A. and Shelton, J. (2005) Understanding the social costs of narcissism: the case of tragedy of the commons. Personality and Social Psychology. 31. 1358–1368.
35. Campbell, W., Foster, C. and Finkel, E. (2002) Does self-love lead to love for others? A story of narcissistic game playing. Journal of Personality and Social Psychology. 83. 340–354.
36. Thich Nhat Hanh (1992) Peace is every step. New York, NY: Bantam.
37. Langer, E. (1990) Mindfulness. New York, NY: Perseus.
38. Heidegger, M. (1927, translated 1962) Being and time. London: SCM Press.
39. Blattner, W. (2007) Heidegger's being and time: a reader's guide. New York, NY: Continuum.
40. Gilbert, D. (2007) Stumbling on happiness. New York, NY: Vintage.
41. Psaris, J. and Lyons. M. (2007) Undefended love. Oakland, CA: New Harbinger Publications.
42. http://www.humanesociety.org/issues/pet_overpopulation/facts/overpopulation_estimates.html.
43. Grogan, J. (2000) Marley and me. New York, NY: Morrow.
44. Kerasote, T. (2008) Merle's door. New York, NY: Mariner.
45. Thompson, M. and Kindlon. D. (2000) Raising cain. New York, NY: Ballantine.
46. Pollock, W. (1999) Real boys. New York, NY: Owl Books.
47. Donovan, J. and Adams, C. (2007) The feminist care tradition in animal ethics. New York, NY: Columbia University Press.
48. Melson, G. (2001) Why the wild things are: Animals in the lives of children. Cambridge, MA: Harvard University Press.
49. Bhikkhu, T. http://www.accesstoinsight.org/lib/authors/thanissaro/notself2.html.

Chapter 6
What Does It Mean to Live an "Extraordinary Life?"

What does it mean to live an "extraordinary" life? Dangerous question for a "recovering narcissist." But this was the question posed to me in November 2008, when I was asked to speak at an event at my home university – Loyola University Chicago. Taking on the task of preparing to give this lecture – to a luncheon crowd composed of students, staff, faculty, and clergy – was an occasion to ponder the ways in which my life of six plus decades might be considered "extraordinary," and so I spent many a walk with my canine companions Hope and Dharma pondering the question.

The obvious, superficial approach to the topic (the narcissistic approach) would be to regurgitate my professional bio, my "curriculum vitae." I have been blessed with a professional career that might be considered "extraordinary," in the sense that I have written more than 20 books, received many professional awards from my colleagues over the years, and have been mentored by some great teachers, like my doctoral advisor and long-term friend psychologist Urie Bronfenbrenner.

This is all good – and even satisfying. But as I walk with Hope and Dharma around the lake I know, of course, that no matter how much awards and publications stoke the ego, they are not really what makes a human life extraordinary. At best they allow me to bask in the glow of accomplishment (a value featured in positive psychology). At worst, they feed the ego, and as a Buddhist Christian, I know that can't be good.

I have also had the opportunity to meet and know some famous people and celebrities along the way. When I participated in the White House "Summit on Youth Violence," in 1999, I shared the day with Bill Clinton and Hillary, Al and Tipper Gore, Attorney General Janet Reno, and singer Gloria Estafan, among others. I have been a guest on "Meet the Press," with Janet Reno, Sen. Joe Lieberman, Pat Buchanan, and Bill Bennet. On a flight from London to Saudi Arabia in 1991, I sat next to ABC News' Ted Koppel, who fell asleep on my shoulder for a couple of hours. When he woke up, I had a chance to talk with him about the differences between being a war correspondent and being a psychologist in a war zone, since we were both on our way to Kuwait in the wake of the Iraqi invasion and withdrawal.

I have shared the stage or television set with people ranging from Mr. Rogers and Captain Kangeroo, to Larry King, Stone Phillips, and Liv Ullman, from Queen Latifah and Bill Maher to Carrot Top and Harry Reems (the male star of the "classic"

J. Garbarino, *The Positive Psychology of Personal Transformation:*
Leveraging Resilience for Life Change, DOI 10.1007/978-1-4419-7744-1_6,
© Springer Science+Business Media, LLC 2011

porno film "Deep Throat"). Once in the same week, I had tea with presidential candidate George McGovern and lunch with Bozo the Clown. And yes, I have appeared on "Oprah." All this was fun, but when I shared these celebrity adventures on with Hope and Dharma, they are unimpressed.

Reflecting on the celebrities I have met on these occasions over the years, I have to agree with Hope and Dharma. This is cool, but not what makes a life extraordinary. Maybe *being* a celebrity would be extraordinary. I can't speak on that. But I do know that simply rubbing shoulders with celebrities isn't enough. Hope and Dharma agree (although Hope seems to think I *am* a bit of celebrity, at least in her life – I take this from the way she gets excited and wags her tail when I enter the room).

Having decided that celebrity encounters are not truly extraordinary, I thought about some of the more unusual experiences I have had during my life, and how they might stack up against my daily lake walks with the dogs. In the southern African country of Mozambique in 1989, at a time when the South African-backed RENAMO insurgency was engaged in destabilizing the country, I was detained briefly by soldiers from the Mozambiquen Army. I was attempting to take what my map suggested was a short cut through the capital city of Maputo, and inadvertently entered an Army base. The fact that I was White and had a map made me a suspicious character, I suppose, and I felt a special dread handing over my passport to the officer in charge – who didn't speak English. After several very tense minutes, someone passed by who spoke English, and through him I was able to explain my purpose – I was actually a guest of the government – and convey my innocence. They let me go, but it did take a while for my heart to return to beating normally.

One night in a Palestinian refugee camp in the West Bank during the Intifada in 1987, my colleagues and I were interviewing families about their experience with traumatic political violence. The father began by explaining the emergency escape route if Israeli soldiers showed up in the camp while we were there. Later, as we walked over a moonlit hill to sleep in another house, our guide cautioned us to be very quiet because, as he said, "they shoot on sight if you are out after curfew like this." That certainly felt "extraordinary" for an American college professor.

It did also when I was in the capital of Cambodia in 1988 and once again was out after curfew. My two female colleagues and I had visited one of the city's few night clubs after a long day of interview work. Everyone else in the place was either Cambodian or Vietnamese, and there was a lot of pressure on my two colleagues to dance with the men – several of whom offered to trade my colleagues for their own "dates" (using the word loosely, to recognize the fact that most of the young women were probably prostitutes). I guarded my colleagues by dancing with both of them at the same time, trying to exude a proprietary air to discourage the other men on the dance floor.

Time passed quickly, and we found ourselves two miles from our hotel as 9:00 pm came. This presented a problem due to the fact that because of the unstable political situation curfew came with nightfall. Outside the club, two security guards offered to take us back to our hotel on their motor bikes – for a fee, of course. So we piled on (me on one and the two women on the other) for the hair-raising ride though the dark streets.

Then there was the rat who shared a room with me in the hotel in Phnom Penh – which also included open sewage running through the room. We had had another "animal encounter" at a comparable hotel in Thailand earlier in the trip when we were visiting Cambodian refugee camps near the border – which were often shelled from guns inside Cambodia. My two assistants came to my room to ask me to help with an insect in theirs. I agreed and found a very large roach sitting on the floor of their bathroom. With shoe in hand, I entered to dispose of him, whereupon the gigantic bug spread its wings and took flight into the shower. My assistants began to scream (I confess I joined them). After a moment some Danish hippies who were staying at the same hotel appeared at the doorway and asked if they could have some of the drugs that they assumed (incorrectly) we were using.

It was on this same trip that we visited a nongovernmental organization to inter-view the director on what turned out to be her birthday. While we were there, she received as a present a birthday cake sent over by her colleagues from the "Mine Demolition Project." Unexploded land mines were (and still are) a huge problem in Cambodia due to the years of war, and I could only think of that as she started to put a knife into the cake. International travel can lead to some interesting experiences.

Closer to home, I think of the times I have visited prisons around the country to interview inmates facing trial for murder, usually in death penalty cases. Testifying in death penalty cases offers an internship in the destructive consequences that can occur when child abuse, trauma, and deprivation come together in a young life. In case after case, I read the records and conduct the interviews, and in so doing, I come face to face with the tales of trauma – physical, psychological, and sexual abuse, street vio-lence witnessed and suffered from, gangs, drug dealing, oppression, and racism.

Many of my cases are retrials of cases decided years earlier but sent back to the courts after appeals, so some of the defendants have already been convicted and sentenced to death. As a result, I have to go to Death Row for some of the cases. Even visiting is a terrible experience. Some films capture the grim emotional reality of it rather well – two examples being "Dead Man Walking" and the more recent "The Life of David Gayle."

I usually drive out into the countryside to some rural site where the prison is located. I surrender ID, cell phone, and anything that might constitute or hide con-traband. Security is usually intense – having a guard watching every moment. Sometimes the condemned is shackled in front of me in the interview room – hands and feet chained to a post. It's grim.

But the logistics are not what's so hard. What's hard is knowing that I am looking at a dead man ("dead man walking") – unless I and the others involved in the case succeed in court. What is hard is knowing that I will walk out the door into the fresh air in a short time and the man (or woman) in front of me will *never* go through that door (since mostly the options in the trials in which I am involved are death, or at best, life in prison).

But what's really hard is hearing the stories of human lives brought so low. When I asked one man on death row what he had learned from 30 years of life he simply said, "Life sucks." I usually swallow and digest this suffering, but not always. One summer several years ago, when three of my cases were coming to fruition at the same time, I traveled to the death row three times in less than five weeks. After the third visit, I spent the time driving back to the airport to go home sobbing. The weight of the suffering was crushing – and I was "just visiting."

I remember a trip to South Carolina almost a decade ago to interview 42-year-old Roger. Roger was born into a dysfunctional family, and this led to him being removed from home and placed in residential facilities until he was 14. He reported experiencing a classic traumatic experience as a young child – witnessing a murder when he was six or seven years old. He retains a clear visual memory of this experience, but reports no emotional or psychological consequences of it, which given what is known about trauma in young children is indicative not of there being no effects, but of "dissociation" and emotional disconnection.

What is more, he was placed in residential programs at which numerous forms of abuse were occurring – including sexual, physical, and psychological maltreatment. And, during his youth he had numerous violent and potentially traumatic experiences, including being shot at. Yet, when asked to name the "worst thing that happened to you as a child" he cites, "being sent away from home." When asked about the "worst thing you ever saw as a child," he reports witnessing the shooting.

These many early traumatic experiences played an important role in shaping Roger's behavior. They were pivotal in his incarceration at age 17 (after just 3 years out of institutions), his difficulties in prison as a young man, and his involvement in the murder for which he was facing the death penalty. The person before me was a tough 42-year-old man. But inside he carried with him many untreated traumas, traumas he experienced as a young child. In a sense, there is an untreated traumatized child inside this 42-year-old man, and that child's unmet needs have played a powerful role in shaping his experiences and behaviors. I think of this every time I remember that on his chest, Roger has a tattoo depicting the Pink Panther – and the tattooed figure is smiling.

Society was unable or unwilling to protect Roger, the young child, and the consequences have been lethal, as they often are in the case of untreated childhood trauma. It was a heavy load to even hear Roger's life story. But there was a light moment at the end of our time together. Unlike in other prisons, where the defendant has been shackled during the interview or a guard close by, in Roger's case we had our talk unattended, in a classroom of the prison school.

When we finished talking, there was no one there to notify, so we waited for a guard to come along so that I could leave and Roger could go back to his cell. As we stood at the doorway waiting, a group touring the prison walked down the hall outside the room – each with a "Hi, I'm...." name tag stuck to his or her shirt. As they approached us, they saw me first – dressed in casual work attire – and smiled. Then, they saw Roger – dressed in an orange prison jumpsuit. Seeing him, their smiles disappeared and were replaced with looks that ranged from horror to fearful concern. After they passed, Roger smiled and said to me, "If I could just get me one of those name tags and some clothes I could be out of here!" Not quite true, but an understandable hope from a "dead man walking."

All these experiences felt quite extraordinary at the time they happened, and my heart was beating fast in a mixture of fear and excitement as I recalled them, but this was not really the point of the lecture for which I was preparing when I began this process of reflection that day in November 2008, in Chicago at Loyola University's lakeshore campus. Being a Jesuit institution, Loyola is very much concerned with "The Big Questions," and when we ask questions like "what makes a life extraordinary," the unstated premise is that by "extraordinary" it meant something tied to living a life guided by spirituality and a commitment to social justice. My experiences around the world began to touch on those issues and were much more significant than my "cool" celebrity encounters, but still were not it.

So then I thought about the amazing experiences of parenthood and marriage, the nuts and bolts of my emotional life. Perhaps here is where I would find my extraordinary life. This is not to say that being a parent or being in a committed relationship is extraordinary in a statistical sense, for after all, most adults share these experiences. But becoming a parent is truly an extraordinary experience in my life as it is for most. It is not simply a matter of light-hearted happiness, of course.

As Daniel Gilbert reminds us, marital satisfaction declines when children are born, and does not recover fully until the last child leaves home. As he puts it, "Every parent knows that children are a lot of work – a lot of really hard work – and although parenting has many rewarding moments, the vast majority of its moments involve dull and selfless eservice to people who will take decades to become even begrudgingly grateful for what we are doing" (p. 244) [1]. But this is precisely what makes parenthood so extraordinary. It offers us an opportunity to engage in some of the most meaningful "work" a human being can do, and everyone knows that important work is not superficially easy and happy-go-lucky. I visit prisons, for heaven's sake, and so I know that parenting is so meaningful because it is so tough *and* so worthwhile. I wrote earlier about the birth of my daughter, so let me recall the birth of my son, Josh, in 1976.

Josh arrived on precisely the date he was due – November 1. There was some fear that he would come the day before – indeed his mother (my first wife Nan) showed signs of going into labor during the early evening – and have the dubious distinction of being a Halloween baby. I was a bit haunted by the possibility because I had a childhood friend who had born on Halloween, and with his orange hair and freckles, he bore an uncanny resemblance to a pumpkin. This was not something I wished for my child, so I was relieved when his mother did not give birth on October 31. But, no sooner had we gone to bed that night and the calendar turned to November 1, Nan woke me up to inform me that "this is it," and off we went to the hospital.

Josh was born that morning – at about 7:00. I was there and the first to hold him when the obstetrical team handed him over. I fed him his first bottle shortly afterward as well. A bit later, while he and his mother slept, I went home to walk the dog – Jacob – and start calling the grandparents. It was an extraordinary experience. As most parents will attest, it is difficult to find the words to adequately describe the experience, the mind-blowing character of becoming a parent.

I had been present and Nan awake throughout the birth (due to diligence in attending Lamaze classes and practicing faithfully during weeks leading up to the big day). This added a special dimension of intensity to the experience, something I became fully aware of when I showed pictures of the birth to the women in my office at Father Flanagan's Boys Town (where I worked at the time as a researcher). All of these women were mothers, yet because of birth practices at the time, *none* of them had been aware at the time their children were born. Each of them had been anaesthetized and thus not really "present" at the birth. To boot, none of their husbands had been in attendance as I had. I felt very fortunate that my son was born where and when he was for that reason (though I think he still holds a bit of a grudge for having been born in Omaha, Nebraska, rather than someplace more hip).

Birth was just the first of the many experiences that nominate being a parent as a critical experience in living an extraordinary life. In the days, months, years, and decades to come, there were many more extraordinary but at the same time, very normal experiences. What can duplicate the horror of discovering that your baby is sick? Josh was jaundiced and had to stay in the hospital for a few days after his mother came home. What can approximate the terror of being responsible for the baby the first night home, when it strains credulity to believe he will breathe on his own the whole night and be alive in the morning? Of course, Josh didn't sleep through the night for an eternally long time after he came home (the calendar says weeks but I find that hard to believe).

Is there any joy like seeing your baby's first genuine, authentic smile? His first successful step? His first recognizable word? His first photo with grandparents? His first day in preschool? His first saxophone lesson? His first swim? His first walk along the ocean? His first date? His high-school graduation, followed, by what sometimes seems like moments later, his graduation from college? His marriage? His swearing into the Illinois Bar after law school?

And what of the horrors, the worries, the fear. The first night his mother and I were away from him for a few hours while he was in the care of a babysitter? The time he nearly drowned? The time he nearly fell off an observation tower at a bird sanctuary? The time he was in a car accident? When he did not pass the Bar exam on the first try?

Anyone who is paying attention can appreciate the wonders of child development, but the special bond between parent and child goes much further. I have taught child development to three decades worth of college students, but nothing is the same as *being* a parent. The Russian novelist Leo Tolstoy captured the uniqueness of the parental perspective in this passage from his epic *War and Peace* in which a mother muses on the extraordinariness of parenthood:

> The universal experience of the ages, showing that children grow from the cradle to manhood, did not exist for the Countess. The growth of her son had been for her at every stage as extraordinary as though millions and millions of men had not already developed in the same way. Just as twenty years before it had seemed unconceivable that the little creature lying under her heart would ever cry, nurse at the breast, or talk, so now she could not believe this same little creature could be that strange brave officer, that paragon of sons and men, which judging by his letter he now was (pp. 291–292) [2].

The wonder and terrors of being a parent are indeed extraordinary, in the most normal of ways. And perhaps that is the true starting point to recognizing an extraordinary life. It is not being a President or a King or a Rock Star or being inducted into some Hall of Fame that defines extraordinariness in a human life. It is living, living aware.

Consider the case of the "Elephant Man," John Merrick. Living in England in the latter part of the nineteenth century, Merrick was the victim of a severe case of neurofibromatosis, in which his entire body was misshapen and covered with large discolored tumors. That grotesque body hid his beautiful spirit and fine mind; therefore, he had to struggle daily to achieve recognition of his very personhood, a fact symbolized by him being called "The Elephant Man." Decades later, anthropologist Ashley Montague offered the following assessment of how Merrick responded when he was befriended and cared for after years of exploitation and rejection as a "freak":

> Merrick bore with courage and dignity the hideous deformities and other ills with which he was afflicted. The nightmare existence he had led during the greater part of his life, he put behind him. He never complained or spoke unkindly of those who had maltreated him. His suffering, like a cleansing fire, seems to have brought him nearer to that human condition in which all the nonessentials of life having fallen away, only the essential goodness of man remained.

Montague, p. 78 [3]

John Merrick's friend and physician, John Treves, wrote this of Merrick: "As a specimen of humanity, Merrick was ignoble and repulsive; but the spirit of Merrick, if it could be seen in the form of the living, would assume the figure of an upstanding and heroic man, smooth browed and clean of limb, with eyes that flashed undaunted courage." (cited in Montague, 1979, p. 37) [3].

What does it mean to be human? Intelligence? Language? Future orientation? Soul? Research on nonhuman primates and dolphins forces the issue. Apes can now communicate with people via sign language and symbolic computerized machinery. Dolphin language is being subjected to sophisticated analysis. Some say that if the intelligence of the planet's organisms were viewed as a landscape, we would readily acknowledge two peaks towering above the hills and plains below. On one would be human beings, on the other dolphins [4]. Hope and Dharma argue to have at least a hill for dogs.

The astrophysicist Carl Sagan looked at the research on the intelligence and language of apes and was led to ask how far chimpanzees would have to go in demonstrating their abilities to reason, feel, and communicate before we define killing one as murder, and before missionaries will seek to convert them. After visiting a lab in which chimps were kept imprisoned in their cages, Sagan wondered: "If they are 'only' animals, if they are beasts which abstract not, then my comparison is a piece of sentimental foolishness…but I think it is certainly worthwhile to raise the question: why, exactly, all over the civilized world, in virtually every major city, are apes in prison" (pp. 120–121) [4].

Why indeed? In the more than three decades since Sagan asked the question, more and more humans are beginning to see the legitimacy of this question – and the many others that arise when we consider the meaning of *human* nature and its differentiation from the nature of the other beings with whom we share the planet. I have no clear and unambiguous answers myself. I know that whenever we assert boundaries and limitations of "the other," we run the risk of prematurely closing ourselves to expanding realities, including realities about core issues in what it means to be human in the world.

Research from modern neuroscience is increasingly documenting the fact that humans can and do experience consciousness beyond what can be explained by the biological circuits of the brain. In their book *The Spiritual Brain: A Neuroscientist's Case for the Existence of the Soul*, Mario Beauregard and Denyse O'leary [5] marshal scientific evidence to document the fact that meditation can change mental experience, that extrasensory perception is real, and that intuition can be a human competence. As they write, "Evidence supports the view that individuals who have religious, spiritual, or mystical experiences do in fact contact an objectively real 'force' that exists outside themselves."

One of the most dramatic illustrations of this expanded understanding of consciousness comes in a report contained in physician/healer Rachel Naomi Remen's book "Kitchen Table Wisdom," [6] a book I received as a gift from my wise friend Donald Gault soon after I learned that I was facing the serious heart condition with which I began this book that appeared to require open heart surgery.

Remen's book charts her course in understanding the processes of healing beyond what she was taught in medical school. Toward the end of her account of this journey, she offers the following story about a man who for the last 10 years of his life had suffered from Alzheimer's disease. As he reached the terminal stage, he could not speak or care for his person in any way, becoming a "sort of walking vegetable." On his last living afternoon as his two adult sons sat with him, the old man slumped forward and fell to the floor – his breath uneven and rasping, his color gray. One of the sons moved to call 911, and as he attempted to do so, their father spoke to them in his "normal voice," not heard in 10 years, saying, "Don't call 911, son. Tell your mother that I love her. Tell her that I am all right." And then he died. One of his sons is himself a cardiologist, and he reported to Remen, "Because he died unexpectedly at home, the law required that we have an autopsy. My father's brain was almost entirely destroyed by this disease. For many years I have asked myself, 'Who spoke?' I have never found even the slightest help from any medical textbook. I am no closer to knowing things now than I was then, but carrying this question with me reminds me of something important, something I do not want to forget. Much of life can never be explained but only witnessed." (Remen, pp. 300–301) [6]. *I know this to be true even while my academically trained mind resists it.* But there is more.

We are not alone in this process of living beyond the limits of conventional knowledge, in living truly extraordinary lives. Let me return to Hope and Dharma, who seem to live beyond the world that I "know" to be true as a twenty-first century "normal" person versed in social science and the humanities. How do they demonstrate a world beyond the obvious limits of the material world? It starts with the observation that dogs manifest "psychic" connections with human beings that go beyond their ability to read our gestures and body language (an ability that is amazing enough on its surface).

This psychic ability has been the focus of biologist Rupert Sheldrake's work on *Dogs That Know When Their Owners Are Coming Home* [7]. Claire reports that when I am returning home after a trip and arrive at the airport, an hour's drive from our home, Dharma knows that my arrival is imminent because he begins a ritual that includes moving to a special place in the house where he can watch the front door (something he only does on these occasions). How does he know? Perhaps he is reading Claire's face or voice and detects some clues in her demeanor that tips him off, but perhaps not. Sheldrake's research suggests not.

Sheldrake and his colleagues [7] have undertaken rigorous studies designed to give dogs (and to a lesser degree other animals including cats) a chance to demonstrate their psychic abilities – mostly in connection with knowing when their owners are returning home from a trip or in finding their owners or homes when they are separated by great distances beyond which smell and sight could offer them enough cues for navigation. Sheldrake's work demonstrates that dogs do have the ability to make use of the energy connections between them and their owners over long distances. He hypothesizes the existence of what he calls "morphic fields" and the ability of dogs (and humans too) to sense these fields and follow their directional flow ("morphic resonance"). It is extraordinary.

Recently, Claire spent half an hour fruitlessly but intently searching for her gloves – being observed all the time by Dharma. Disappointed after all the effort, we left our house and walked out into the cold. When we returned three hours later, there sat the gloves – in the middle of the hall, at Dharma's feet. Coincidence? We don't think so. Did he understand the word "glove" and appreciate through hearing her words that she was looking for them? We don't think so (although he does know a lot of words, we have never seen evidence before or since then that "glove" is one of them). We think that as Claire so intently focused on her gloves, the image was "out there" to be retrieved by the dog (who demonstrates other aspects of a highly developed sensitivity, including Sheldrake's morphic resonance).

Having retrieved the image of the gloves, he proceeded to retrieve the gloves themselves – either coincidently as he prowled the house in our absence and "discovered" the missing gloves, or intentionally as he recalled their location and sought them out. The intersection of modern neuroscience and the experience of sensitive people who live with sensitive dogs lead me to believe that human and canine beings can perhaps connect psychically.

Hope demonstrates similar sensitivities, mostly about detecting the presence of other dogs walking by our house even when the windows are closed, the wind is blowing away from our house, and the other dog is silent. She also does this when we silently open a package containing a favorite food when she is outside, well beyond any hearing or smelling range. She does this particularly if Dharma is near the food and she is not. All these abilities of dogs – and humans – seem impossible to many whose perspective is fixed by the tenets of conventional science. For them, these abilities are impossible.

But by the same token, it was once thought (less than 100 years ago) that it was impossible for a human being to run a mile in less than 4 min. Now it is done regularly at elite track meets. *Once the idea of its impossibility was discarded, a new reality emerged.* To a normal person of the eighteenth century, the concept of radio waves, television, cell phones, and wireless internet-connected laptop computers would have seemed preposterous (unless you were Jules Verne, of course) [8].

Beyond the problem of cultural conceptions and personal preconceptions that limit our ability to see what humans (and dogs and other animals) can do is the fact that all too often researchers and other observers attempt to draw conclusions about the competence of both humans and dogs by assessing them in situations that do not allow what competence they do have to express itself. For example, the famous Swiss psychologist Jean Piaget [9] concluded from his limited observations that young children cannot take the perspective of others. Later researchers found that children can accomplish this task if it is presented to them in contexts with which they are familiar.

Some researchers in the 1950s concluded that African-American children were verbally impoverished, even mute, on the basis of observing them in a strange and presumably intimidating laboratory situation in which White strangers asked them questions. Other researchers found these same children were extremely vocal when tested by an African-American interviewer in a familiar situation in which they felt comfortable [10].

Human development books and articles of the past are littered with assertions about what people can and cannot do that have fallen by the wayside as the next generation of researchers devise situations that permit people to express their competence. "Performance in a particular situation does not necessarily demonstrate the limits of competence" is an important principle in modern efforts to understand human development [11]. I hope we will choose to live by this as a society.

Who knows what contemporary "facts" of psychology will become obsolete in the future? Perhaps many of the common diagnoses and "disabling disabilities" of today's psychology and psychiatry will prove to be as unsubstantial as sand castles in the face of the advancing tide as our understanding of brain development and neural modification proceeds. One need only to read Norman Doidge's book *The Brain that Changes Itself* [12] to find numerous example of brain-related diagnoses that were once thought to be permanent in adults but have been shown to be subject to modification through neural retraining, including stroke-related damage, ADD, obsessive-compulsive disorder, and phantom limb pain syndrome.

When it comes to the competence of dogs, we must always remember that canines – like human beings – are social beings, pack animals. That is the context in which they evolved their many competencies – particularly their acute sensitivity to facial expressions and body language and their use of these capacities to communicate. In this they are unlike solitary pandas, for example, who have little use for such sophisticated communication and thus have evolved faces that are noticeably expressionless. And they are unlike chimpanzees, who are not attuned to human gestures and, unlike dogs, cannot make use of human pointing to gain access to things they want (like food hidden under a covering bowl) [13].

The special nature of the human–dog relationship is that dogs have evolved to include us in their pack, to allow us into their inner circle in which the group is all, and have even gone beyond their wolf ancestors in developing special competence in "reading" human beings and presenting themselves in ways that elicit human care – for example, their life-long baby-faced quality (the technical term for which is "neoteny"). But this does not mean that dogs have given up their essential natures and characteristics, only that they have adapted them to the world they share with people.

It should come as no surprise then that their ability to recognize themselves should be demonstrated in a social situation (as I recounted back in the first chapter of this book). The point of their being is precisely to exist as part of relationships – with humans and with other dogs. They don't stand alone. Even a "lone wolf" is defined by his separation from his pack, a separation that he seeks to end by finding a mate and establishing a new pack. An individual wolf hardly exists without reference to the social group.

Interestingly enough, human infants likewise do not exist apart from social relationship. As the great psychoanalyst Donald Winnicott [14] put it: "There is no such thing as a baby," meaning that to survive and develop, a human infant must be in relationship with caring others. This is indisputable in the early months and years of life on a physical basis but is also true and continues to be true on an emotional and cognitive level as the child grows up. Indeed, as cardiologist Dean Ornish [15] has found in his research on preventing and reversing heart disease, social isolation is a powerful negative influence on human health, including cardiac health. Like dogs, humans thrive in relationship, not in isolation.

Russian psychologist Lev Vygotsky [16] recognized that to develop, children need relationships (preferably relationships with humans more sophisticated than they are so that these individuals might serve as teachers). Children without relationships become intellectually and emotionally stunted – if they survive at all. Research suggests a mechanism for the destructive effects of social isolation: it undermines the immune system and depresses motivation. And these effects extend to the critical issue of identity development. This may be hard to see for those of us who live in an individualistic culture, but it rings true nonetheless.

Human cultures differ with respect to the level of individuation expected and encouraged. Most traditional cultures (and even some modern ones) are collective in the sense that identity is mostly a social phenomenon: "I am defined by who we are." Modern individualistic American culture is unusual in this respect historically and cross-culturally. And it is not surprising that social isolation is such a powerful issue in our society, since the very idea of individuals existing separate from the group runs against the human grain.

Many observers have noted this – for example, David Riesman in his 1950 classic book *The Lonely Crowd* [17]. Recent research on "happiness" documents this as well – noting, for example, that one reason why Danes are happier than Americans is that Danish society supports and encourages the primacy of relationships, while American society promotes the competitive pursuit of material affluence (and the avoidance of poverty) ahead of cultivating relationships [18]. Social connection is the cornerstone of Tal Ben-Shahar's best-selling book *Happier: Learn the Secrets of Daily Joy and Lasting Fulfillment* [19]. What do humans want? If we have our wits about us, the answer is the same as it is for dogs: we want others of our kind. Wise humans don't see the same human/animal boundaries that the less attuned among us see, and therefore, they want dogs as much as they want "other" people, others of their own kind.

Perhaps helping us to recognize the primacy of social connection for experiencing durable happiness and confident identity is one of the services that dogs can offer to human beings, particularly American human beings growing up in our pathologically individualistic culture. Living with dogs offers an affirmation of social solidarity as the basis for identity. It helps adults put first things first – and we all benefit from that clarification of priorities. Dogs can stabilize families, and this works to our advantage in recognizing what is most important about human life – connection with the living presences that surround and infuse us. What is most important? Showing up! And having the wisdom to pay attention.

The wise Zen Buddhist monk and teacher Thich Nhat Hanh says it so well when he tells us that the miracle is not walking on water, it is walking on the Earth [19]. He intends no Christian blasphemy, but simply to make it clear that being alive is a miracle – as any parent knows. *It is the ordinary opportunity of life that is the beginning and the ending point of the quest to assess the extraordinary in any life.* The miracle *is* to walk the Earth and to be fully aware and appreciative of that opportunity.

It's not easy. In her powerful memoir *The Spiral Staircase*, Karen Armstrong [20] said it well after seven years in a convent trying to become a Christian nun and years more seeking to find her way in the academic world. As she feels happy without condition in a rare moment of serenity one evening she reports: "As T. S. Eliot has noted: 'time is always time. And place is always and only place.' This was all we had. But that night, for once, I was wholly present in the moment, not looking before or after, or pining for what was not. And the present moment was not a bad place to be." (p. 191) Indeed, it is the best and only place to be!

Providing inspiration to do so is one of the functions of art and music. Writing of the Marlboro music summer program – in which some of the most talented, indeed extraordinary, young musicians come to rustic Vermont to perfect their craft and embed themselves in the fellowship of equally talented peers and mentors, Alex Ross [21] says this: "Marlboro is an enchanting place, but, in the end, there is nothing especially remarkable about it. The remarkable thing is the power of music to put down roots wherever it goes." (p. 65) This is the appreciation of miracles I seek, and which figures importantly in a positive psychology of being human.

And once again, dogs can play a role in helping us to appreciate the miracle of walking the Earth, even in their dying. The stories of their lives are intertwined with ours, and because their biological clocks tick faster than ours, to walk with them usually means to witness their deaths. I know this when I walk with Hope and Dharma. As we saw from my daughter Joanna's 14-year relationship with her dog Abby recounted earlier, the potential of dogs' deaths for teaching life lessons is enormous.

Chief among these lessons is the fundamental paradox of faith: attachment to self is the surest way to unhappiness; giving up control and trusting is the gateway to happiness. With a mind that had been trained to distrust itself and with the daily challenge of living with epilepsy, Karen Armstrong said it well: "It would be a lifelong task, requiring alert attention to the smallest detail, dedication and unremitting effort; but as I listened…that day, I knew it could be done. My confidence sprang from the fact that the process had already started. I had resolved to stop fighting my malady, to accept what my life had become, and – 'consequently' – for the first time in years I had responded spontaneously and with my whole being to a poem, just as I had before I incurred this damage. It was a sign of life, a shoot that had suddenly broken through the frozen earth." (p. 142) [20]. Her conclusion is mine as well: "This must be the way that human life worked. He who loves his life shall lose it; he who loses his life shall save it. This was not an arbitrary command of God, but simply a law of the human condition." (p. 142) Not so much faith in God, but faith in life.

It has been more than 60 years since I began to walk the Earth, and blessings continue to accrue. Almost a year after my atrial fibrillation was diagnosed, my heart returned to a normal rhythm – to the surprise of my cardiologist. A year later I faced a cancer scare, but the biopsy came back normal. Visiting the death-row prison in South Carolina in connection with a new case, I had an occasion to reunite with Roger, who I had interviewed four years before, and once again be impressed with the sweetness of the abused child who lives within him.

I saw "Avatar" four times, and developed a crush on the 10-foot tall blue Na'vi woman Neytiri on the planet Pandora. Hope, Dharma, and I started walking some of the time in a new location because a friend offered access to her 100 acres of wooded trails. Claire and I continue to deal with the ups and downs of our relationship. And I continue to discover opportunities for expanding my circle of caring.

On May 17, 2010, I arrived in El Salvador as faculty advisor for a group of undergraduate students from Loyola University, to begin a nine-day Immersion Program organized by International Partners in Mission (IPM). The terrible violence and trauma of life in El Salvador during the political oppression and civil war of the 1970s and 1980s, and the subsequent gang violence that came to plague the country were very much on our minds those nine days we spent traveling around the country. How could it not be as we visited sites at which religious and political activists were assassinated, and where innocent civilians – mostly women and children – were massacred?

But I arrived for that immersion program with El Salvador already very much on my mind and weighing heavily on my heart. I had just begun work on a new case, a case that had its roots in El Salvador. Alfredo Prieto stands convicted of murders both in California and Virginia, but he started his life in El Salvador. Born in 1965, his childhood was marked by domestic violence in his family, and savagely disrupted by the political violence of the 1970s. His mother left him behind to seek work in the USA, leaving him in the care of his older siblings and other family members. As a child and a teenager, he witnessed acts of grotesque traumatic violence – beheadings, shootings, beatings. His grandfather was assassinated in front of his eyes when the boy was 15, and with this, his mother came back to El Salvador to bring him with her to the USA. Living as a poor, fatherless immigrant in Los Angeles, he promptly joined Pomona North Side – one of the Hispanic gangs that were dominating the immigrant community and engaging in a reign of violence and drug dealing. Out of this terrible developmental cauldron, he emerged as a killer, and eventually I was asked to serve as an expert witness in his case.

The violence that dominated Alfredo Prieto's childhood did not end with the Salvadoran Peace Accords that brought a formal end to the civil war in 1992. By 2010, in El Salvador the political violence of the 1980s had been replaced by gang violence – in part because of the actions of demobilized soldiers and rebels who were trained in violence but little else, in part because of the 34,000 Salvadoran gang members who had been deported from the USA back to El Salvador, and in part because of the crushing poverty and illiteracy that affect communities all over the country.

Every American should feel a special responsibility for these developments because it was our tax money that funded the political oppression of the 1980s (to the tune of a million dollars a day) in military aid to a government that engaged in massacres of its citizens and repression of anyone who dared to speak up for social justice on behalf of the poor and disenfranchised – like Archbishop Romero in 1980, and the six Jesuit priests who were killed in 1989. And it was our tax money that funded the US Army's School of the Americas that trained the military officers who led the repression and ordered the massacres. It is not just McDonald's and Kentucky Fried Chicken that we have exported to El Salvador and the rest of Central America.

How does all this history relate to the experience the students and I had as participants in the IPM Immersion in May 2010? We were all struggling to figure out how all this fit together every day of our trip, until the second-to-last day, when we visited the Lidia Coggiola School – a project supported by IPM in the El Zaite area of Zaragoza, a community of great poverty and gang domination.

After introducing ourselves to the children, the students and I sat down with the children to undertake a craft project. When I had finished with my group, I sat on the floor with my back against a low cinder-block wall to watch the children and the students having a great time together. While I sat there, a little girl came up to me, sat down in my lap, and snuggled up against me. It was a blissful moment. I sang her a lullaby, and we sat together until the activity was over and the kids were herded off to their classrooms by the teachers.

How did the life of Alfredo Prieto connect with the lives of Salvadoran children now, and this little girl in particular? As a psychologist who has spent his professional life focusing on issues of abuse, violence, and trauma, I knew that young children are rarely as ready as this child was to seek comfort in the arms of a stranger unless they were victims of abuse and neglect at home or in some other way have been traumatized. So, rather than just seeing this little girl as just a particularly friendly child, I was alerted immediately to the likelihood that her behavior was a sign of loss rather than just cuddliness. The school's Director Carlos Diaz confirmed this. Her father is a gang member who drinks, does drugs, and abuses the little girl and her mother. Although more than four decades separated their births, Alfredo Prieto and this little girl were both abused in their families and neglected by their societies.

In a flash I knew what I had to do. I had to find a way to make some small gesture to help close the circle of caring, to make amends somehow for my sense of American responsibility for what happened in El Salvador while my death penalty case client was growing up. At lunch a few minutes after our experience with the children, I learned that the school had a program to promote literacy among the children – and their parents (some 60% of whom are illiterate). "Do you have a library?" I asked. "No," replied the Carlos. "I want to donate the money to create a library for the children in the school, a library that can support your literacy program," I replied.

At that moment I knew that through this small gesture I could make a small start toward completing the circle of caring in my heart by donating the money that

I would be earning as an expert witness in the Prieto case to the school. Although this small individual act may be insignificant in the big picture, I feel that "returning" this money to El Salvador is a tiny step toward helping to close the circle of caring that was ruptured decades ago.

We can't change what happened to Alfredo Prieto as a boy four decades ago, but we can perhaps exert some small positive influence on the life of the little abused girl who snuggled in my lap, and the other children around her who struggle with life today in Zaite, El Salvador. What a blessing it is to have an opportunity through IPM to make a small contribution to closing the circle of caring in this way. Recognizing and welcoming these opportunities for grace is crucial to experiencing the extraordinary life in front of me – indeed in front of each of us.

It has been more than 60 years since I began to walk the Earth, and I know I am still taking baby first steps to be fully aware of this opportunity. That I have any inkling of this is what is extraordinary about my life. Walking with Hope and Dharma I know this. For them it is obvious. The joy of the smells and sounds and sights of the forest, the pleasure of their company with each other and with me are crystal clear in them. We walk together. They wag their tails. And if I had a tail to wag, I would join them in the tail wagging. I don't, so the best I can do is smile – and wear the shirt I often wear when I walk them that says "life is good." Or maybe it is better to say "living is good." Whichever it is, it's quite extraordinary.

References

1. Gilbert, D. (2007) Stumbling on happiness. New York, NY: Vintage.
2. Tolstoy, L. (2010; 1923) War and peace. New York, NY: Nabu Press.
3. Montague, A. (1979) The elephant man. Lafayette, LA: Acadian House.
4. Sagan, C. (1986) The dragons of Eden: Speculation on the evolution of human intelligence. New York, NY: Ballantine Books.
5. Beauregard, M. and O'leary, D. (2008) The spiritual brain: A neuroscientist's case for the existence of the soul. New York, NY: HarperOne.
6. Remen, R. (1997) Kitchen table wisdom. New York, NY: Riverhead Trade.
7. Sheldrake, R. (2007) Dogs that know when their owners are coming home. New York, NY: Three Rivers Press.
8. Verne, J. The complete Jules Verne collection. Amazon Digital Services, Kindle Edition.
9. Piaget, J. (2001) The psychology of intelligence. New York, NY: Rutledge.
10. Labov, W. (1963) The social stratification of English in New York City. New York, NY: Cambridge University Press.
11. McClelland, D. C. (1973) Testing for competence rather than "intelligence." American Psychologist. 28, 1–13.
12. Doidge, N. (2007) The brain that changes itself. New York, NY: Penguin.
13. Hare, B., Brown, M., Williamson, C., and Tomasello, M. (2002) The domestication of social cognition in dogs. Science. 298, 1634–1636.
14. Winnicott, D. (1964) The child, the family and the outside world. Harmondsworth, England: Penguin Books.
15. Ornish, D. (1995) Dr. Dean Ornish's program for reversing heart disease. New York, NY: Ivy Books.
16. Vygotsky, L. and Kozulin, A. (1986) Thought and language. Cambridge, MA: MIT Press.

17. Riesman, D. (1965) The lonely crowd. New Haven, CT: Yale University Press.
18. http://www.pbs.org/thisemotionallife/topic/connecting/staying-connected.
19. Ben-Shahar, T. (2007) Happier: Learn the secrets of daily joy and lasting fulfillment. New York, NY: McGraw Hill.
20. Armstrong, K. (2005) The spiral staircase: My climb out of darkness. New York, NY: Anchor.
21. Ross, A. (2009) Onward and upward with the arts, the "music mountain." The New Yorker. June 29, p. 56ff.

Index

A
American Psychiatric Association
  homosexual humans, 36
  sexual orientation, 35, 36
  US military, 35
Asperger's syndrome, 33

B
Biophilia hypothesis, 4, 5
Buddhism, 20, 60, 73, 74, 94, 95, 99

C
Child development
  acceptance vs. rejection, 29
  corporal punishment, 37
  empirical studies, 69
  psychological malignancy, 29
  sexual orientation, 36
  social conventions, 27
  stable marriages, 29
Christianity, 68, 73, 74, 94

E
Enlightenment
  Dharma, 1–3, 5, 11, 12, 19
  consciousness, 4
  dogs
    abuse of, 10
    acute depression, 13
    archeological research, 14
    biological characteristics, 16
    canine traits, 16
    communication, 2
    cultural conception, 10
    early warning system, 15
    genetic research, 14

happiness interventions, 13
instinctive morality, 5
mechanical behaviors, 10
moral development, 7
Neanderthals, 15
norm of sharing, 6
self-identity, 17
unfair treatment, 5
Hope, 1–3, 5, 11, 78
humans
  abnormal personality development, 10
  autism, 13
  awareness, 4
  behavioral habits, 3
  biochemical reactions, 4
  child–canine relationships, 11
  cultural and psychological models, 8
  dogfights, 11
  institutionalized cruelty, 10
  interaction and stimulation, 17
  literary treatment of dogs, 9
  moral responsibility, 7
  positive psychology, 12
  prosocial behavior, 8
  shelter dogs, 9
  spiritual equality, 4
  women's right, 4
  transformational experience, 4
  Zen teacher, 20
Extraordinary life
  art and music, 114
  child development, 108
  dolphin language, 109
  emotional/psychological consequences, 106
  energy connections, 111
  human cultures, 113
  human–dog relationship, 112
  identity development, 113
  international travel, 105

Extraordinary life (*cont.*)
   literacy program, 116
   modern neuroscience, 110
   parenthood, 108
   performance, 112
   political violence, 115
   psychic ability, 110
   social isolation, 113
   social justice, 107
   traumatic political violence, 104

H
Human evolution. *See* Biophilia
       hypothesis
Humanistic psychology, 18
Humanities, 68, 69, 72, 73
Human studies
   autobiography, 72
   intersubjective transmissibility, 72
   soul searching, 73
   subjective experience, 72

I
Immunization, 54

N
Narcissism
   Bakan's analysis, 82
   biological determinism, 87
   Buddhism, 95
   confronting death, 98
   consumers, 91
   culture, 88
   emotional expressiveness, 97
   existentialism, 94
   healthy human development, 91
   human development, 94
   mental-health professionals, 84
   parental acceptance and rejection, 87
   personality disorder, 85
   positive psychology, 93
   psychological health, 86
   rational self-interest, 92
   secure attachment, 81
   self-aware altruism, 84
   self-esteem, 85
   social justice, 99
   social skills training, 90
   temperamental risk factors, 89
   total absorption, 93

O
Obama, Barack, 1, 9
Obliviousness
   acceptance *vs.* rejection, 29
   annihilation, 37
   baby boomers, 23
   childhood, positive psychology of, 25
   child sexual abuse, 37
   Cuban missile crisis, 38
   cultural equipment, 29
   demographic reality, 23
   developmental assets, 26, 28
   gays and lesbians, 36
   human development, 25
   middle class, 24
   neurological system, 32
   obscure, 33
   positive power, 25
   professional psychological community, 35
   racism, 31
   religious sectarianism, 31
   Search Institute, 27
   self-indulgence, 23
   sexual activity, 27
   social competition, 29
   social environment, 24, 28
   social skills training, 33
   stable marriages, 29
   substance abuse and violence, 27
   television environment, 39
   terrorism, threat of, 38
   traditional American values, 31
   video recording, 39
   youth-related activities, 23

P
Posttraumatic stress disorder (PTSD), 49

R
Resilience. *See* Trauma
Rights of animals, 4
Rights of children, 4

S
Science, 68, 69, 72, 73
Scientists and humanists
   academic psychology, 69
   chaos theory, 65
   empirical studies, 69, 70
   falsifiability, 69

human development, 69, 71
hypotheses, 70
negative psychology, 65
positive psychology, 73
psychoanalysis, 69
reincarnation, 70
soul searching
    overwhelming positive arousal, 75
    spiritual realities, 74
spiritual growth and consciousness, 68
subjective human studies, 66
transformational grace
    acute incidents, 77
    altruism and service, 76
    chronic trauma, 77, 79
    divine opportunities, 77
    mindfulness, practice of, 79
    physical experience, 76
Social toxicity
    annihilation, 37
    communications technologies, 30
    traumatic imagery, 40
    violent television, 39

T
Trauma
    accommodation and assimilation, 50
    automobile crash, 45
    cats, 43
    chronic traumatic danger, 50

compassion, 58
dehumanization, 59
divorce, 44
electric shocks, 52
forgiveness, 58
functional resilience, 57
hardiness, 56
human reactions, 55
human vulnerability, 48
immunizing vs. sensitizing, 54
individual resilience, 56
individual's maladaptation, 52
kindling depression, 54
media technologies, 53
mental-health problems, 54
overwhelming arousal and cognitions, 49
physical violence, 52
plane crash, 45
political violence, 47
psychological threat, 48
psychopathic personalities, 55
self-medicating, 55
social and intellectual resources, 51
social fabric, 52
spiritual transformation, 60
strap explosives, 53
terminal thinking, 61
UNICEF, 47
utter reconcilability, 60
violent crimes, 59
war zones, 51

CPSIA information can be obtained at www.ICGtesting.com
Printed in the USA
LVOW010121170112

264201LV00004B/8/P